D1795323

925 -

Showing, Sensing, and Seeming

Showing, Sensing, and Seeming

Distinctively Sensory Representations and their Contents

Dominic Gregory

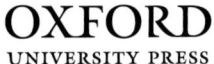

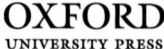

OXFORD
UNIVERSITY PRESS

Great Clarendon Street, Oxford, OX2 6DP,
United Kingdom

Oxford University Press is a department of the University of Oxford.
It furthers the University's objective of excellence in research, scholarship,
and education by publishing worldwide. Oxford is a registered trade mark of
Oxford University Press in the UK and in certain other countries

First Edition published in 2013

Impression: 1

Published in the United States of America by Oxford University Press
198 Madison Avenue, New York, NY 10016, United States of America

British Library Cataloguing in Publication Data
Data available

ISBN 978–0–19–965373–7

As printed and bound by
CPI Group (UK) Ltd, Croydon, CR0 4YY

For Rosanna, Lydia, and Miranda

Preface

This book develops a theoretical framework for studying the contents of all those actual and possible representations that are 'distinctively sensory', in that the representations show things as looking or sounding or otherwise standing sensorily certain ways. (Many pictures are distinctively sensory representations, for instance, as many pictures show things as looking certain ways; the sensory mental images often involved in our imaginings and memories are also distinctively sensory representations.) The book uses the resulting theory of distinctively sensory content to address a varied family of issues relating to distinctively sensory representations of more or less specific kinds.

Chapters 1–3, plus the Introduction, form the core of what follows: the remaining chapters rely heavily upon the theory of distinctively sensory content presented in Chapter 3, whose formulation relies in turn upon ideas developed in the previous chapters and in the Introduction. Each of Chapters 4–8 has a fair degree of autonomy, however. Chapter 4 explores various general issues concerning distinctively sensory contents and shows how the theory developed in Chapters 1–3 may be used to shed light on various forms that distinctively sensory contents may take. Chapters 5–8 examine in detail some restricted varieties of distinctively sensory representations. Some readers may prefer to move straight on to those chapters once they have encountered the theory articulated in Chapter 3.

The ideas contained in this book have gained a great deal from other people's reflections upon them. Most importantly, I have benefited enormously from written and spoken discussions with my friend and colleague Rob Hopkins and with my wife and colleague Rosanna Keefe. Both Rob and Rosanna read most of the material in earlier drafts of this book and they provided me with a great number of sharp, constructive, and insightful comments that hugely affected the book's final form. Rosanna, in particular, has patiently read multiple versions of significant chunks of the book and her comments always helped me significantly to improve it. Two anonymous referees for Oxford University Press (OUP) also supplied very helpful and extensive written comments on an earlier draft. Their advice, criticisms, and questions helped me to overhaul and improve almost all of the manuscript.

Numerous other philosophers have provided me with additional help. Malcolm Budd gave me very useful and encouraging comments on some initial work that I produced on the distinctively visual contents of pictures and visual mental images, in 2007. Many thanks, too, to Chris Hookway for the help which he gave me with the proposal that I submitted to OUP; and many thanks to Penelope Mackie, whose support helped me to get a period of Arts and Humanities Research Council (AHRC)-funded leave in 2007, in which I first started working on the ideas developed below.

I also received some very helpful anonymous referees' reports on various papers arising from my work on distinctively sensory contents. In particular, I am very grateful to anonymous referees for the *British Journal of Aesthetics*, *Mind and Language*, and the *Philosophical Quarterly*. Note that Chapter 6 draws heavily upon Gregory 2010c, a paper published in *Mind and Language*; many thanks to the editors and publisher of that journal (John Wiley and Sons) for allowing me to incorporate material from that paper in this book. Chapter 7 contains a few paragraphs from Gregory 2010b, a paper published in the *British Journal of Aesthetics*; many thanks to that journal's editor and to its publisher (OUP) for allowing me to use the relevant material here.

I received a lot of helpful comments from the audiences at various talks which I have given in recent years. Many thanks, more specifically, to those who attended the departmental seminars that I gave during the last five years at Manchester, Sheffield, and Warwick; to the audiences who attended the talks which I delivered at the 2010 British Society of Aesthetics annual conference and at the 2011 conference on 'Perceptual Memory and Perceptual Imagination' that was organized by Glasgow's Centre for the Study of Perceptual Experience; to those who attended the talks which I gave to Oxford's Jowett Society in 2011 and to the Reading Philosophy Society in 2010; and to the Anglo-German picture theorists who attended a talk which I gave to a meeting of the Anglo-German Bildtheorie/Picture Theory Group in Jena in 2012.

Family and friends have also provided me with helpful comments and advice. Many thanks, in particular, to my parents Ian and Julia Gregory. (It will be no surprise that I was aided by the former, so memorably described by *The Times*'s 'Lawyer of the Week' on 7 March 2013 as '[t]he greatest philosophical and legal mind of the 21st century'; but the latter—whose virtues were justly celebrated in the same article—was a great help too.) Thanks also to my siblings Ben and Tessa; to Terry and Sheila Keefe, and to Simon Keefe and Celia Hurwitz-Keefe; to Sophie Hannah and Dan Jones; and to Hamish Cunningham.

I was lucky enough to receive generous amounts of leave during the period in which this book was written, without which it would never have seen the light of day. I have been very well treated by two bodies: first, Sheffield's philosophy department; and, second, the Arts and Humanities Research Council. I first started working on this book during the 2007–8 academic year, the first half of which I spent on departmental research leave and the second half of which I spent on leave that was funded by the AHRC's Research Leave scheme. I then spent the 2010–11 academic year on a period of leave that was funded by the AHRC's Early Career Fellowship scheme; and I spent the latter half of the 2011–12 academic year on departmental leave. I am hugely grateful both to the AHRC and to the Sheffield philosophy department for their support.

I am also very thankful indeed to Peter Momtchiloff at OUP, both for his practical editorial advice and for his encouragement, and also to Eleanor Collins at OUP for all her help with seeing the book into print. I also wish wholeheartedly to thank NASA (for Figure 4.3), the Victoria and Albert Museum (for numerous figures in the text), and the Kimbell Art Museum (for the image used on the cover), three organizations whose unusually enlightened attitude towards the use of their images in academic publications both provided me with ideal pictures for various purposes and saved me a fortune in licensing costs.

Contents

List of Figures   xii

   Introduction   1
1. Things to Explain   14
2. Matters of Perspective   27
3. A Theory of Distinctively Sensory Content   45
4. Applications and Extensions   70
5. Mental Images   98
6. Pictures   130
7. More on Pictures   157
8. Distinctively Sensory Records   184
   Conclusion   212

References   217
Index   225

List of Figures

2.1 The Müller-Lyer illusion   28

4.1 'Poor Gaudy Butterfly': caricature of Arthur Lennard (1905),
George Cooke   72

4.2 Old man (perhaps Tobit) reading to a seated woman (seventeenth
century), copy after Rembrandt van Rijn   75

4.3 The 'Eskimo' Nebula (NGC 2392), NASA A. Fruchter and the
ERO Team (STScl)   78

4.4 The Temptation and the Expulsion from Paradise, after
Michelangelo's fresco in the Sistine Chapel (eighteenth century),
Domenico Cunego   81

4.5 Seated figure of a man (late seventeenth–early eighteenth century),
Jean-Antoine Watteau   84

5.1 A map of a fictional island; from Kosslyn, Ball, and Reiser 1978   103

5.2 Some pairs of drawings; based on original images included in
Shepard and Metzler 1971   104

6.1 A rabbit, by a toddler   135

7.1 Interior of Antwerp Cathedral (c.1640), Pieter Neefs (the elder)   158

7.2 Cushion cover panel (1904), The Silver Studio (designer)   162

7.3 Watercolour—Tulips (after 1668), Simon (Pieterz.) Verelst   164

7.4 The Resting Horseman (1640s), Louis Le Nain   178

8.1 Miranda and Lydia eating cupcakes (2010), Rosanna Keefe   186

Introduction

A type of representations

Visualize a table. Your visual mental image—taken strictly on its own, without any accompanying mental patter—only informs you about certain properties of the table that you have imagined. The image may show the table as having a shiny surface, for example, but it does not show you the total history of the materials from which the table's surface was made.[1] That is because the image's portrayal of a table derives from the way that it shows things as looking. And the total history of the matter from which a table is made is not something that is made apparent to one merely in the way that a table looks.

Your visual mental image of a table characterized the table by showing things as looking a certain way. But visual mental images obviously are not the only representations which show things as looking certain ways. Photographs may show how things looked in specific past circumstances, for example, and illustrations in novels may show how things look in fictional situations. Films may also show things as looking a series of ways from a single place at a series of times; or they may show things as looking a series of ways from a changing series of places.

Just as visual mental images do not provide the only examples of representations which show things as looking certain ways, so representations which show things as looking certain ways do not provide the only examples of representations that are especially sensory in the general

---

[1] It might be objected that visual mental images are not really even capable of displaying tables; rather, visual mental images are like vision itself in merely having to do with, say, 'colour, light and shade, shape, size, motion, and spatial relations' (Armstrong 1962, 5). My apparent assumption that visual mental images can literally show tables is merely an expository convenience, however, a point that is explored briefly in this Introduction and at more length in Chapter 4.

fashion illustrated by visual mental images, pictures, and the rest. Auditory mental images show things as sounding certain ways, for instance, and we sometimes interpret playbacks of audio recordings as sonic analogues of moving pictures. ('Sometimes', because we do not always treat playbacks in a representational manner; we often regard them more straightforwardly, merely as sounds that we hear.) Tactile mental images show things as feeling certain ways; olfactory mental images show things as smelling certain ways; and gustatory mental images show things as tasting certain ways.

More generally, suppose that we are given some sensory modalities. (The relevant modes of sensing might be drawn from the traditional five human senses of sight, hearing, smell, taste, and touch, but they might not be. I shall count our immediate kinaesthetic awareness as sensory, for example; and I will allow for sorts of sensations which humans do not experience, like the echolocatory sensations famously enjoyed by bats.) And suppose that we are given a representation which stands to those sensory modalities as, say, visual mental images stand to vision. Suppose, that is, that we are given a representation which does some showing that is bound to the given sensory modalities, just as visual mental images, in showing things as looking certain ways, thereby do some showing which is tied to vision. Then the representation is *distinctively sensory*.

The class of distinctively sensory representations encompasses many cases which differ pretty radically from one another. It includes sensory mental images plus many pictures and playbacks of audio recordings, for instance. But it seems that there is a level at which the class's members are alike, and at which they are different from many other representations: just intuitively, none of the sentences on this page 'shows' things as looking or sounding or smelling or otherwise standing sensorily certain ways. What makes distinctively sensory representations like one another and different from representations of other sorts?

This book uses some fairly humdrum thoughts about sensory mental images, suitable pictures, and other kinds of distinctively sensory representations as the basis for a theory concerning their *contents*. It then uses the resulting theory to address a wide spread of intellectual problems. Some of the issues discussed concern distinctively sensory representations in general, but others relate to distinctively sensory representations of more specific sorts. (Sensory mental images, pictures, photographs, and memories are all examined below, for instance.) The theory thus receives support on two fronts: on the one hand, from its status as a relatively sophisticated and illuminating elaboration of simpler things which we already believe; and, on the other, from its usefulness in further theorizing.[2]

According to the approach developed in detail below, the characteristic contents of distinctively sensory representations are alike in two crucial ways. First, they single out types of sensations in a special 'subjectively informative' manner. I hold that the special way in which the representations' contents pick out types of sensations is what accounts for the fact that the representations 'show' things as standing sensorily certain ways. And, second, the contents use the types of sensations thus singled out either to characterize sensations or to characterize what things are like around perspectives. (The two options isolated in the previous sentence will allow us to account for two fundamentally different kinds of distinctively sensory representations that are initially identified in the next chapter.)

To summarize the theory, then, using a couple of captions whose import will become clearer in Chapter 3:

Distinctively sensory showing comes from subjective informativeness. And *distinctively sensory representations show things as standing sensorily certain ways, either from perspectives or in sensations.*

Chapters 1–4 form the book's first part. Chapter 1 isolates some important general facts about distinctively sensory representations, facts that ought to be explained by any satisfactory theory of the representations' contents. Its discussions rely on our pretheoretical sense that there are significant differences between those representations which show things as standing sensorily certain ways and those representations which do not show things as standing sensorily certain ways. Chapter 1 therefore does not attempt to

---

[2] It is very common for the justificatory support for philosophical theories to work in this dual fashion. To take a related philosophical example, part of the case for possible worlds semantics (as elaborated in Lewis 1973 and 1986, for instance) cites its status as a relatively sophisticated and illuminating refinement of some of our ordinary ways of expressing modal claims. (People commonly say that 'there is a possibility that such-and-such' when they wish to state that such-and-such is possible; similarly, possible worlds semantics offers 'there is a possible world at which such-and-such' as an analysis of 'it is possible that such-and-such'.) But the case for possible worlds semantics also derives from the further theoretical utility of the framework; from, for example, its ability to reduce the inferential relationships between many modal claims to the inferential relationships between claims which quantify over possible worlds.

provide a theoretical account of, say, what makes for the difference between 'showing' things as looking some way and just 'describing' what things look like; that task is saved for Chapter 3.

Chapter 2 surveys some important background material relating to sensations, types of sensations, and perspectives. Various ideas from that chapter will play an important role in Chapter 3's eventual account of one of the two fundamental kinds of distinctively sensory contents. Chapter 2 also introduces some resources relating to particular sensory modalities which will be useful in later chapters.

Chapter 3 presents the book's general account of the nature of the contents of distinctively sensory representations. It also provides some initial illustrations of the account's power, by showing how the theory may be used to explain the general features of distinctively sensory representations described in Chapter 1. Chapter 4 discusses a range of more concrete examples in the light of the framework presented in Chapter 3, with the aims of dramatizing the flexibility of the resulting approach and of resolving some general issues which might seem to present difficulties for it. The chapter also examines some general theoretical issues about the status of distinctively sensory contents, by drawing upon Chapter 3's account of the relationships between distinctively sensory contents and sensory states proper.

Chapters 5–8 then employ the views spelled out in Chapters 1–4 to address numerous questions relating to more specific groups of distinctively sensory representations. Chapter 5 examines sensory mental imagery, while Chapters 6 and 7 discuss pictures. One common thread running through Chapters 5 and 6 is the thought that, by invoking theoretical assumptions concerning what is special about the contents possessed by distinctively sensory representations, we may shed light upon the special ways in which distinctively sensory representations couched in different media express their contents. Chapter 8 illustrates how the concepts and arguments developed in the previous chapters may be brought to bear upon some further philosophical issues, by exploring the nature of 'distinctively sensory records', a type which encompasses many memories along with photographs and analogous non-visual phenomena.

As remarked already, there are very many possible types of distinctively sensory representations. Indeed, the following pages have considered only a fairly small selection of the sorts of cases which we actually encounter. There are no discussions of sculpture below, for instance, yet

I think that many sculptures are rightly regarded as being distinctively sensory representations. But why think that the group of distinctively sensory representations is of any more philosophical interest than other, randomly thrown-together, bunches of representations? And just which representations are distinctively sensory? Does live theatre count, say?

The full theoretical interest of the class of distinctively sensory representations is not really visible at this point, even though the idea that it possesses an overall unity is plausible enough at first glance. The class's importance should become clearer further down the line, however, once the general framework to be developed below is in place; just as the full theoretical importance and unity of, say, the class of birds—as opposed to the class of birds plus flying mammals, insects, and other airborne fauna—only becomes fully apparent in the light of fairly elaborate biological ideas. Later parts of this book will demonstrate that our untutored sense that something important unites all those representations which show things as standing sensorily certain ways does in fact reflect deep underlying relationships holding among the representations.

The reader will look in vain, though, for a handy test to decide whether any given representation is distinctively sensory. This book's investigations are, in the first place, driven by the evident connections that exist among various striking cases like sensory mental images, suitable pictures, and appropriate playbacks of audio recordings. And they are guided by the thought that the naturalness of describing all of those cases as representations which show things as standing sensorily certain ways indicates the presence of a common nature that is worth sounding out. A theoretical description of that shared nature is then offered and used for various tasks.

The theory's application to the representations which most clearly show things as standing sensorily certain ways is most straightforward, as one would expect. Its applicability to phenomena which are less evidently classifiable as distinctively sensory representations—like, say, live theatre and opera—is less clear, again as one would expect. More generally, the precise reach of the theoretical framework is a matter for further debate. And the debate will need to be informed by reflection upon the particularities of the bewildering variety of examples which seem somehow to be interestingly related to the cases that provide the theory's initial impetus.

Theorizing about content

One of the main contentions of this book is that the contents of distinctively sensory representations are alike in certain important respects; and one of the book's main tasks is to provide a theoretical account of the ways in which the contents of distinctively sensory representations are alike. The result of that enterprise will be a 'theory of content' of a specific sort. To clear the way for all that, it will be worth saying a little about theories of content in general and theories of distinctively sensory content in particular, to differentiate such theories from theories of related but importantly different kinds.

Consider the following sentence:

(I.A)   Water boils at 100°C.

We may identify (I.A)'s content—what is grasped by anyone who understands (I.A), merely on account of the person's understanding of the sentence—with a certain proposition P.

In the wake of Kripke's famous discussions of natural kind terms,[3] it would commonly be claimed that P has certain features. More specifically, many would hold that the truth-value possessed by P relative to an arbitrary possible situation depends upon whether the specific stuff H_2O vaporizes at 100°C in that situation. (The truth-value of P relative to a possible situation does not then simply depend upon whether the clear drinkable liquid which there happens to fill the seas and rivers, and which more generally plays there the roles which H_2O plays in our world, boils at 100°C; P relates essentially to H_2O.)

Those last claims solely concerned the nature of the content which belongs to (I.A). In particular, none of the statements bore immediately upon how it is that (I.A) comes to have its content. None of the claims directly said anything concerning how the use of the term 'water' in (I.A) might result in that sentence's expressing a proposition that is essentially about the particular substance H_2O, for instance. Nor did any of the claims say anything about how the brutely physical properties of (I.A), like the shapes of the sentence's letters and the order in which those letters

---

[3] See, for example, relevant parts of Kripke 1981.

were placed, might combine with facts about our wider environments to make us associate the specific proposition *P* with the sentence. But one may seek theories which address those concerns. Thus many philosophers, again following Kripke, are inclined to think that the referential properties of natural kind terms and proper names are generally determined by their transmission along chains of communication that start with suitable ostensive or descriptive 'baptisms' and whose links are connected by intentions to co-refer.[4] And maybe the distinctive role which such chains of communication play in enabling us to understand natural kind terms somehow also ensures that (I.A) expresses a proposition which is essentially about H_2O.

It is important to note, though, that we have here distinct types of issues, ones which call for theories of different sorts. We have, on the one hand, questions pertaining simply to the nature of the content expressed by (I.A): for example, the question whether the proposition expressed by (I.A) is in fact essentially about H_2O. And we have, on the other hand, questions which involve (I.A)'s content but which involve other matters as well: questions about how it is that (I.A) comes to possess whatever content it possesses, for example, or questions about how we manage to understand (I.A).

Theories which exclusively address questions of the former sort—that is, ones which restrict themselves to claims concerning the nature of the contents which belong to certain representations—are *theories of content*.

To return to the earlier example, Kripke engaged in some very influential theorizing about content. In particular, his thesis that sentences which use the term 'water' express propositions that are essentially about H_2O forms part of an important theory of content for natural kind terms. But Kripke's philosophical enquiries also led him away from theorizing about content. In particular, his thesis that the referential properties of natural kind terms are typically the products of their transmission along chains of communication cannot form part of a theory of content. That last claim concerns *how* certain representations come to possess their contents; it therefore does not simply concern the nature of the contents which the representations possess.

---

[4] See, for example, Kripke 1981, 96.

Theories of distinctively sensory content

The totality of what is represented by a distinctively sensory representation is often rather complicated. Allegorical paintings may communicate abstract ideas, for instance, and portraits may show how things looked on specific past occasions. Yet there is, in those cases, an especially basic layer of information which may be recoverable even by one who fails either to access the relevant abstract ideas or to identify correctly the relevant past occasions. For a person who fails in those respects—and who hasn't?—may nonetheless grasp the ways that the relevant pictures show things as looking; and the person may appreciate what the pictures thereby represent.

Someone might use a picture to show me how things once looked to some unidentified individual, for instance; or someone might use a picture to show me what things were once like around some unidentified place. In either case, I may grasp what the relevant unidentified sensation or place is meant to be like, by appreciating the ways that the pictures show things as looking. My appreciations of the ways that the representations show things as looking have then led me to an awareness of certain properties that appropriate items are characterized as possessing, without leading me to identify any specific things as being characterized as having the relevant properties. (Parallel phenomena evidently arise in relation to linguistic representations. You may understand what my assertion that Nyirimana is a boy says 'about someone' without being aware of who Nyirimana actually is.)

With the exception of Chapter 8, this book's discussions of the contents of distinctively sensory representations will be entirely concerned with the foregoing particularly elementary layer of their contents. That is, the book will largely focus upon those aspects of the contents of distinctively sensory representations that derive merely from the ways that the representations show things as standing sensorily. I will therefore commit the peccadillo of sometimes speaking as though *all* that distinctively sensory representations represent is the stuff which they represent on account of the ways that they show things as standing sensorily.

Even with the foregoing restriction in force, though, additional questions may come swiftly to mind. Did your earlier visual mental image 'of a table' really represent *a table* by virtue of showing things as looking a certain way, for instance? Or was its content more primitive than that? It might be suspected that tables as such feature neither in the ways that things literally look to us to be, nor in the ways that visual mental images literally show things as looking. Rather, it might be suggested, we sometimes seem to see scenes including variously coloured surfaces at certain distances; and we then use our conceptual capacities to categorize the items thereby apparently seen as tables, chairs, and the like.

I will not attempt definitively to resolve those issues in this book; the theory of distinctively sensory content articulated below passes the buck on them, as Chapters 3 and 4 will make clear. The account entails, for instance, that pictures and visual mental images are able to represent tables as such—that is, as falling under the concept *table*—only if visual sensations may involve apparent encounters with tables presented as such. More generally, the theory entails that the answers to many hard questions about distinctively sensory contents depend upon the answers to correspondingly tough questions about the ways that things may seem to be to sensing subjects. But the theory does not itself pretend to settle the latter questions.

The theory's resulting neutrality on a wide range of problematic philosophical topics is a virtue, as it makes the theory consistent with a wide range of philosophical starting points.[5] Of course, the theory's neutrality would be problematic if it prevented the theory from having any useful applications. But, as we will see below, it does not have that consequence. For the connections which the theory posits between distinctively sensory contents and sensory states are themselves sufficient for many significant philosophical tasks. Anyway, I will generally continue to speak as though familiar items like tables and chairs may be represented as such by distinctively sensory representations, just for convenience's sake.

Suppose that you are investigating some distinctively sensory representations—a group of pictures, say. You might try to develop a theory of content for the relevant pictures. More precisely, you might attempt to describe the nature of the particularly primitive layer of the pictures' contents distinguished at the start of this section: you might try to describe the nature of the contents which the pictures possess on account of their

---

[5] To return to an analogue employed in an earlier footnote, philosophical and logical uses of possible worlds semantics are able to proceed pretty far without engaging in any metaphysical controversies concerning what possible worlds are really like (see Gregory 2006 for more on that point).

showing things as looking certain ways. But you might also engage in some content-related theorizing about the pictures which is not simply theorizing about content. Suppose, in particular, that you argue that we grasp the ways that the pictures show things as looking on the basis of what the pictures themselves look like.

Imagine that you eventually broaden your attention, so that you come to be concerned with the family of distinctively sensory representations as a whole. Your theory of pictorial content might promise to generalize, to provide a theory of distinctively sensory content per se. But your vision-based account of how we grasp the ways that pictures show things as looking will struggle to generalize to a comparable degree. For how could it smoothly be extended to cover those distinctively sensory representations—like, say, sensory mental images—which we do not encounter using our senses at all?

There is, more generally, an important form of abstraction which looks to be available to us if we concentrate upon constructing theories of distinctively sensory content. For the idea that we can give a uniform account of the special nature of the contents of all those representations which show things as standing sensorily certain ways seems quite plausible.[6] But the relevant kind of abstraction looks harder to attain if we focus upon the widely varied mechanisms by means of which we grasp the contents of families of distinctively sensory representations.

There are other respects, too, in which theories of distinctively sensory content might provide a nice generality. The truth of sentence (I.B) below ensures the truth of sentence (I.C):

(I.B)   Lydia and Miranda are sisters.
(I.C)   Lydia has a sister.

Similarly, the truth of (I.D) ensures the truth of (I.E):

---

[6] Note that a theory of distinctively sensory content which implies that, say, pictures and visual mental images are alike in having distinctively sensory contents of an especially visual sort does not also have to imply that, for any visual mental image, there can be a picture which possesses the very same distinctively sensory content; nor need it imply that, for any picture which shows things as looking certain ways, there can be a visual mental image which has the very same distinctively sensory content. In particular, the theory of distinctively sensory content articulated in this book is compatible with the view—with which I agree—that the nature of the media called upon by some variety of distinctively sensory representations may affect the nature of the distinctively sensory contents which can belong to representations of the relevant kind.

(I.D)   Lydia et Miranda sont soeurs.

(I.E)   Lydia a une soeur.

It is no accident that the implicational relationship holding between (I.B) and (I.C) is mirrored by that holding between (I.D) and (I.E): there is a proposition *P* and a proposition *Q* such that (I.B) and (I.D) express *P*, where (I.C) and (I.E) express *Q*; and the truth of *P* entails the truth of *Q*. That example illustrates how we may sometimes provide unified explanations of related facts about disparate representations, by invoking relationships among the contents which the representations express; this fact is a cornerstone of logical enquiry.

To take a distinctively sensory case, it seems to be no coincidence that both pictures and visual mental images of tables cannot, merely by showing things as looking certain ways, thereby show the total history of the materials from which the displayed tables were made. One might consequently hope to provide an explanation of that common representational restriction which relies solely upon assumptions concerning the nature of the contents possessed by representations which show things as looking certain ways. More generally, then, theories of distinctively sensory content promise to provide explanations which bring under one roof numerous phenomena involving distinctively sensory representations of very different kinds.

Finally, note that theories of content are basically theories of aspects of information, where that last term is construed in a colloquial sense: they are accounts of the different sorts of materials that can form part of what is learned, communicated, known, believed, supposed . . . So, reconsider sentence (I.A) above ('Water boils at 100°C'). And suppose that the content of that sentence is proposition *P*, where *P* is essentially about H_2O, as Kripke claims. Then one would expect *P* to crop up in the course of further theorizing about situations from which the sentence (I.A) itself is absent.

A visitor to earth might soon learn by observation that water boils at 100°C, for example, without ever having encountered sentence (I.A). But *P*—the content of sentence (I.A)—is therefore able to play an important role in good descriptions of the ways in which experience of our world has affected the alien's knowledge. For *P is* the information which the alien has newly acquired. Kripke's theory of content for natural kind terms then tells us that the information acquired by the alien, which may form part of the alien's subsequent thoughts and reasonings, is essentially about H_2O. Theories of content thus have the power to expand our horizons in a way that few other enterprises can hope to do, by telling us more about the very stuff of cognition.

Of course, some theories of content may be more philosophically interesting than others, because some types of information are philosophically more significant than others. Theoretical accounts of the special nature of contents relating to fairground rides are likely to be less valuable for philosophical purposes than theoretical accounts of the special nature of contents relating to moral value. But the aspects of information corresponding to the contents of distinctively sensory representations are certainly important ones. Our lives are soaked in comprehending encounters with representations which show things as standing sensorily certain ways—just consider sensory mental images and pictures—and the importance to human affairs of the aspects of information corresponding to the contents of distinctively sensory representations would be hard to overestimate.

Restricted types of distinctively sensory representations have been intensively studied in many different ways, and we will encounter the fruits of some of those efforts later in this book. But there is, to my knowledge, nothing which has previously tried to provide a theory of distinctively sensory content in general, for all the points just made.[7] Chapters 1–4

---

[7] The exploratory work by Husserl posthumously collected in Husserl [1898–1925] 2005 has a generality which is analogous to that displayed by the current book. Husserl's phenomenological ideas about distinctively sensory representations are quite different from the theory of distinctively sensory content developed here, however. Walton suggests that we should 'broaden our understanding of "depiction" to include representations that are auditory or tactile or otherwise perceptual in the way that paintings are visual' (1990, 296). But Walton's own treatment of the resulting category—as determined by his statement that '[a] *depiction*, then, is a representation whose function is to serve as a prop in reasonably rich and vivid perceptual games of make-believe' (1990, 296)—very sharply differentiates it from the category of distinctively sensory representations. (The visual mental images which accompany many of our memories show things as looking certain ways, for example, but they are not props in Walton's perceptual games of make-believe.) As one of this book's referees noted, some of Haugeland's ideas concerning the representational genus of 'iconic representations'— a genus which he seeks to identify in terms of the nature of the contents belonging to the genus's instances (1998, 184–5)—come closer to the broad approach to be developed here. But Haugeland's class of iconic representations is clearly distinct from the class of distinctively sensory representations. In particular, the contents of the former—which 'might be conceived as variations of values along certain dimensions with respect to locations in certain other dimensions' as illustrated by, say, the information supplied by a graph tracking an object's

undertake that task; the remainder of the book puts the resulting ideas to work.

The exclusive focus of this book's first part upon theorizing about content, in combination with its focus upon the class of distinctively sensory representations as a whole, thus marks it out by comparison with the extant literature on types of distinctively sensory representations. So, we will see in Chapter 6 that philosophers have recently constructed accounts of how pictures depict things; but those theories are very different from the theory of distinctively sensory content developed below. Similarly, and as we will see in Chapter 5, the last few decades have spawned a massive literature concerning the representational format of the mental representations underlying visualizations; those theories are, again, very different from this book's theory of distinctively sensory content.

As we will also see in those chapters and elsewhere, however, the previous contrasts certainly do not mean that the theorizing about distinctively sensory content undertaken below has no relevance to earlier work. In particular, reflection upon the theory's application to specific ranges of distinctively sensory representations like sensory mental images and suitable pictures yields important conclusions about how representations of those kinds may express their distinctively sensory contents. While the theory of distinctively sensory content presented later will be used in plenty of pure theorizing about content, then, it will also be used to generate lots of arguments bearing upon distinctively sensory representations in other respects.

temperature over time (see p. 192 for both the quotation and the example)—lack the special sensoriness which is essential to distinctively sensory contents.

1

Things to Explain

The Introduction grouped together an enormous range of actual and merely possible representations under a common heading. The resulting family of 'distinctively sensory representations' encompasses all those representations which show things as standing sensorily certain ways. Pictures that show things as looking certain ways are distinctively sensory representations, for example, as are olfactory mental images; while films that show things as looking and sounding certain ways are distinctively sensory representations too.

The project of explaining in detail what unifies the class of distinctively sensory representations will be undertaken in Chapter 3. But if there really is an interesting unity here, one would expect it to be manifested by more superficial similarities that are symptomatic of the deeper likeness. The current chapter identifies some illustrative examples of properties which distinctively sensory representations seem to possess on account of the distinctively sensory nature of their contents.

The relevant characteristics provide striking points of contrast between distinctively sensory representations and representations of other familiar sorts. They thus form a set of symptoms which reinforce our intuitive sense that distinctively sensory representations are alike at some suitably abstract level.[1] I take it that the properties identified in this chapter are also features of distinctively sensory representations which ought to be explained by any decent theory of distinctively sensory content. Chapter 3 provides explanations of them all using the theory of distinctively sensory content formulated there.

The current chapter also distinguishes two significantly different types of distinctively sensory representations: 'subjective' ones, which represent

---

[1] The list of general properties singled out in this chapter corresponds to part of a list of properties of pictures examined in Hopkins 1998.

sensations, and 'objective' ones, which do not. We seem commonly to encounter both subjective and objective distinctively sensory representations and it is natural to think that theories of distinctively sensory content ought to explain how there can be distinctively sensory representations of both sorts. The theory of distinctively sensory content presented in Chapter 3 will meet that demand.

Perspectivalness

Visualize a chair. Your visual mental image shows a chair from a certain perspective. To quote Peacocke, visualizing 'always involves imagining from the inside a certain (type of) viewpoint, and someone with that viewpoint could, in the imagined world, knowledgeably judge "*I'm* thus-and-so", where the thus-and-so gives details of the viewpoint'.[2]

Similar points apply to other types of distinctively visual representations. Consider a portrait of somebody. The picture will show the person in a perspectival manner; perhaps it shows its subject from the front.[3] More generally, the perspectival nature of the showings of worldly items and scenes performed by distinctively visual representations mirrors the perspectival nature of vision: what we seem to see, we seem to see from some perspective.

The perspectival natures of sensations of other sorts are likewise reflected by their corresponding types of distinctively sensory representations. Use auditory mental imagery to imagine your mother calling to you. Your imagery presents the imagined voice in relation to a perspective, just as the experience of seeming to hear a voice situates the voice in relation to an implicitly defined perspective. Your auditory mental image may have shown[4] a voice as coming from the left, say, or from all around;

---

[2] Peacocke 1985, 21.

[3] The perspectivalness of picturing is a commonplace in the literature on pictorial representation: see, for example, Budd 1993, 169–70; and Hopkins 1998, 27. Note that there is no implication in the text that a given distinctively sensory representation may show a certain item from just one perspective. More generally, the theory of distinctively sensory content developed in this chapter allows for multiperspectival distinctively sensory contents, as it needs to; see Chapters 4 and 7 for discussion of some pertinent cases.

[4] Talk of 'showing' things comes most naturally to us in relation to distinctively visual representations like pictures and visual images, and it is prone to sound somewhat clumsy in relation to, for instance, auditory mental images and playbacks of audio recordings. I take it, though, that there is a special sort of representational relationship in which, say, auditory

or—to gesture at another kind of case that should be familiar to users of headphones—it may have placed the voice 'dead centre'.

It is easy enough to provide examples which illustrate the link between the perspectivalness of various sensory modalities and the perspectivalness of their corresponding types of distinctively sensory representations. It is harder to articulate precisely the relevant general concept of perspectivalness. But I will save until Chapter 2 further discussion which bears on that general idea. For it is equally hard to conceive of any sensory modality that is perspectival and whose perspectivalness does not generate a corresponding perspectivalness in its corresponding range of distinctively sensory representations, in roughly the sort of manner illustrated by the previous examples—whatever exactly that all comes to.[5]

The perspectival aspects of distinctively sensory representations just considered provide an obvious contrast with some other types of representations. So, a verbal description of a village ('Barmby Moor is a notable village in the East Riding of Yorkshire. It has a long and noble history; it was once a market town with a coaching inn . . .') need not represent the village 'from somewhere'. And some non-verbal representations are not perspectival; it is easy to produce non-verbal and non-perspectival Venn diagrams, for instance.

Sensibilia

The fifteenth-century Italian polymath Alberti famously stated that 'the painter is concerned solely with representing what can be seen',[6] a

---

mental images stand to those items which the representations represent by virtue of the ways that they show things as sounding, where distinctively visual representations stand in the same relationship—a relationship which we there naturally call 'showing'—to those items which they represent by virtue of the ways that the representations show things as looking. My talk about the items that are 'shown' by distinctively sensory representations just provides a handy formula for talking about that relationship.

[5] Note that I am not assuming that every possible sensory modality is perspectival in the way that, say, vision is perspectival. The phenomenon identified in the text is a conditional one: if a certain sensory modality is perspectival—in the sense that apparent encounters with things by means of the modality situate the items in relation to a perspective—then any distinctively sensory representation whose content is bound to the relevant sensory modality will show whatever items it shows in a correspondingly perspectival manner. (In particular, if there are sensory modalities which do not generate sensory appearances, those sensory modalities will not be perspectival in the relevant sense; and the theory developed below implies that their corresponding forms of distinctively sensory representations also will not be analogously perspectival.)

[6] Alberti [1435–6] 1966, 43.

comment which has often been echoed: Lessing also claimed that 'bodies with their visible properties are the peculiar subjects of painting',[7] for instance, while Picasso spoke slightingly of those painters who, poisoned by 'the spirit of research', had sought to 'paint the invisible and, therefore, the unpaintable'.[8]

An initial point: suppose that there is some property whose presence cannot in fact be visually detected, although it can look to us like the property is instantiated. (Some of the properties whose instantiations we apparently encounter in visual illusions, like the 'moving but staying still' which makes the Waterfall Illusion so striking, are perhaps like this.[9]) Then maybe someone could make a picture showing an instantiation of the property.

Alberti's talk of 'what can be seen' therefore needs to be read so that his comment amounts to the following: 'the painter is concerned solely with representing what can *apparently* be seen'. And the distinctively sensory nature of pictures—those which show things as looking certain ways, anyway[10]—is surely what explains the preceding constraint. Anything which represents a scene by showing things as looking some way will struggle thereby to represent aspects of the situation which could not look to be there. Given all that, though, one would expect non-visual distinctively sensory representations to be subject to analogous handicaps.

And they are. Use kinaesthetic mental imagery to imagine a flexing of your left arm. That imagery displays a particular series of bodily movements by showing things as feeling certain ways. But everything which the imagery thereby represents is the sort of thing which one could seem to sense through one's kinaesthetic powers. Or consider a playback of an audio recording, where that playback captures how things once sounded from a certain window near a beach. The playback may thereby present various events—children shouting, birds singing, waves rolling in . . . — but everything that it does thereby represent will be something which one could seem to hear.

---

[7] Lessing [1766] 2005, 91.
[8] Fry 1966, 166. There have been apparently dissenting voices: Klee stated, for example, that '[a]rt does not reproduce the visible but makes visible' (Klee 1961, 76).
[9] See Crane 1988 for further discussion.
[10] I think that there are representational pictures which do not show things as looking certain ways; see Chapter 6.

More generally, take some distinctively sensory representation. The range of items which the representation shows, and the range of properties which the representation shows the things as having, will be limited in a crucial respect: if the representation shows an *F* as being *G*, a subject could seem to encounter an *F* which is *G* by means of the sensory faculties involved in the ways that the representation shows things as standing sensorily. And this representational restriction directly mirrors the nature of our sensory capacities themselves; we can seem to see only what we can seem to see, for example.

The constraints noted here are evidently ones which differentiate distinctively sensory representations from representations of some other varieties. We can, for instance, easily use language in purporting to describe denizens of the outside world which we could not seem to sense.

Relative specificity

Another interesting group of restrictions on the powers of distinctively sensory representations reflect respects in which the ways that things may seem to us to be, in the course of sensory episodes, sometimes operate at relatively high levels of specificity.[11] Suppose, for example, that you seem to see a red ball, a yellow ball, and a blue ball standing in a horizontal line. Then the red ball will either look to be on the left or look to be on the right; the red ball will not just look to you to be *either* on the right *or* the left.[12]

Similar points apply elsewhere. Any auditory sensation in which a ringing is apparently heard will not merely thereby involve the apparent presence of a ringing that has 'some pitch'. Rather, the pitch of the apparent ringing will fall within a relatively narrowly circumscribed

---

[11] Dretske's examination of 'analog and digital coding' in Chapter 6 of Dretske 1981 incorporates some discussion of this sort of phenomenon (the next example in the main text is adapted from Dretske 1981, 137–8); see also Hopkins 1998, 24–7, for an examination of the following phenomenon as it applies to pictures. The cases that I am about to introduce deploy particular assumptions about our sensory powers that may turn out to be false. But the details of the examples are not important. What matters is that the reader can derive from the examples a sense of the general connections that they are meant to exemplify, along with an appreciation of how the putative connections cited would place distinctively sensory representations under corresponding constraints.

[12] Section 3 of Heck 2007 uses the sorts of points made above to argue that visual sensations involve contents that are, in a sense, non-conceptual.

region. More generally, then, it is sometimes the case that, when we are apparently confronted in sensations by things having features which enable us to place the items under fairly general concepts, the apparently sensed items must seem sensorily to us to be items of comparatively more specific varieties.

That observation is not very precise but it is nonetheless sharp enough to indicate a significant aspect of distinctively sensory representations, one which seems to arise from their distinctively sensory status. For they too are sometimes forced to characterize the things which they show as being of relatively determinate types.

Transformations of recent examples may be used to illustrate that last point. Consider a picture which shows 'a yellow ball . . . situated between a red and a blue ball',[13] where the balls are in a horizontal line. Then '[e]ither the blue or the red ball must be pictured on the left'.[14] Or consider a playback of an audio recording, one which shows things as sounding certain ringing ways. The playback will thereby supply some relatively specific information about the pitches of the various ringings; it will not merely characterize the ringings as 'having pitch'.

More generally, suppose that we are given a distinctively sensory representation whose content is bound to some sensory modality. And suppose that the representation shows an item as having some features which enable us to place it under a fairly general concept C. Finally, assume that the following holds: any sensory episode falling under the relevant modality, in which we apparently encounter an item having properties which enable its categorization as falling under C, must amount to an apparent encounter with something of a comparatively more specific type. Then the representation's showing of an item which falls under C must likewise amount to the showing of something of a comparatively more specific type.

The general restriction just noted supplies further clear contrasts between distinctively sensory representations and representations of some other sorts. A mere verbal description of a yellow ball as placed in a

---

[13] Dretske 1981, 137.
[14] Dretske 1981, 138. Dretske himself stresses the parallel between sensation and picturing illustrated here; he writes that '[s]ensation, what the ordinary man refers to as the look (sound, smell, etc.) of things, and what the psychologist refers to as the percept or (in some contexts) the sensory information story (SIS), is informationally profuse and specific in the way a picture is' (1981, 142).

horizontal line between a red ball and a blue one does not settle which of the latter two balls is on the left, for example. Nor is it difficult for us to talk about ringings as having pitch without saying any more about their pitches. This section and the preceding ones catalogued some very general representational limitations to which distinctively sensory representations are subject on account of their distinctively sensory nature. The relevant limitations ought to be explained by any satisfactory theory of distinctively sensory content. I offer explanations of the constraints in Chapter 3. The resulting explanations illustrate how this book's theory of distinctively sensory content is in fact able to account for a much wider variety of related representational constraints that apply to distinctively sensory representations.

The next section distinguishes two fundamentally different types of distinctively sensory representations—'subjective' and 'objective' ones— both of which seem at first glance to be unproblematic. But I will then present a simple argument which purports to demonstrate the impossibility of objective distinctively sensory representations. The chapter concludes by sketching a line of response to the argument. The sketched response contains the germ of a way of accounting for the difference between subjective and objective distinctively sensory representations, by suggesting a way of differentiating between two modes of 'showing things as standing sensorily certain ways'.

Chapter 3 takes the hint; the theory of distinctively sensory content developed there incorporates the suggested modal distinction, using ideas worked out in the next chapter. When the resulting theory is combined with various ancillary premisses—premisses which are not essential to this book's theory of distinctively sensory content but which have, I hope, wide appeal—we will be able to explain how both objective and subjective distinctively sensory representations are possible.

Subjective and objective

Consider a picture of a table. It seems clear that the picture need not represent 'from the inside' a visual encounter with a table: the picture could show a table without thereby representing the table *as seen*. More generally, it seems clear that the picture need not represent any sensations at all. Similarly, it seems that a visualization of a table need not involve an imagined seeing of the table—nor need it involve any other imagined sensations. Analogous points apply to distinctively sensory representations whose contents are bound to non-visual modes of sensation. Playbacks of audio recordings, for example, can represent events by showing how they sounded, without thereby characterizing the events as overheard.

Our apparent ability to produce distinctively sensory representations which do not represent sensations provides a point of contact with our sensations themselves. If one seems to see a table, for instance, one does not seem to see the very subjective episode which is one's apparent seeing of a table; nor does one necessarily seem to see a subjective episode of any other sort. Is one's apparent seeing of the table posited by the visual episode itself in some other manner? An affirmative reply to that question is highly counter-intuitive. Anybody who always ascribes to visual episodes self-referential contents—ones which make those very visual episodes somehow part of what the episodes themselves posit—seems to provide an overly complex account of the nature of visual sensations in general.[15]

Many distinctively sensory representations thus seem to be *objective*, in that they do not represent sensations. But many other distinctively sensory representations appear to be *subjective*. For there seem to be many representations which, in showing things as standing sensorily certain ways, do thereby represent sensations.

As Wollheim notes, for example, '[w]hen I visually imagine, or visualize, an event, there are two modes of doing so. I can imagine the event from no one's standpoint . . . [o]r I can imagine it from the standpoint of one of the participants from the event, whom I then imagine from the inside'.[16] Pictures, too, seem sometimes to show how things look in the course of visual sensations; pictures are sometimes used like that in constructing first-person narratives in comics, for instance. Suppose that a

---

[15] Searle 1983 advocates the view that the 'conditions of satisfaction' of visual sensations make reference to the causal antecedents of those visual sensations themselves (see, for example, p. 48 of Searle's book). I think that Searle's position just conflates the conditions under which the visual appearances involved in a visual sensation are accurate with the conditions under which the relevant visual sensation counts as a genuine seeing. It is worth noting, though, that this book's theory of distinctively sensory content does not itself assume that the contents of our sensations never somehow make reference to the relevant sensations themselves. That assumption is simply invoked in some of my own uses of the theory.

[16] Wollheim 1987, 103.

given distinctively sensory representation represents a sensation from the inside. Then the representation *portrays* the sensation.[17]

It seems, in fact, that the cores of particular objective and subjective distinctively sensory representations may be the same. Visualize a table, for example. Your visual mental image of a table may have been an objective distinctively sensory representation. Yet, even if the visual mental image was an objective distinctively sensory representation, it seems that you could just as easily have used visual mental imagery to portray a visual sensation in which things look the very way that your earlier visual mental image showed things as looking. The resulting visual mental image would then be a subjective counterpart of an objective distinctively sensory representation.

How can that be? How can one visual mental image which shows things as looking a certain way thereby portray a visual sensation, when another visual mental image which shows things as looking the very same way does not portray a visual sensation? For that to be possible, the fashions in which the visual mental images show things as looking a single way must somehow be different. That is, there must be distinct modes of showing things as looking the relevant way. What are those different modes? And what are the relationships between them? I will return to those questions at various points below.

There seem to be both objective and subjective distinctively sensory representations, then. But appearances can be deceptive. The next section presents an argument for thinking that there cannot in fact be objective distinctively sensory representations because distinctively sensory representations must always portray sensations.

---

[17] It is not clear that every subjective distinctively sensory representation must portray a sensation. A distinctively sensory representation is subjective just in case the representation shows things as standing sensorily certain ways and thereby represents a sensation. Now imagine a faculty which involves the apparent sensing of *sensations* and which generates, in particular, a way for things to stand sensorily that meets the following condition: anyone to whom things stand sensorily that way thereby seems to encounter a subject who is, say, seeming to see a chair. Then why couldn't there be a distinctively sensory representation which, in showing things as standing sensorily the former way, just characterizes what things are like around some perspective? If that were to be possible, though, the representation would represent an apparent seeing of a chair, merely by placing an apparent visual encounter with a chair in the outside world rather than by representing from the inside an apparent seeing of a chair, just as photos of chairs may represent chairs simply by placing chairs in the outside world.

'No Lookerless Looks'

Visualize a red light on the left and a green light on the right. The resulting visual mental image represents the red light as being to the left of a perspective, with the green light being to the perspective's right. While the image thus represents a perspective, it does not do this by explicitly showing the perspective; just as a visual mental image may represent a visual sensation from the inside without explicitly showing the visual sensation.

Rather, Martin claims, '[t]he red light is imagined as before and to the left of the point of view within the imagined situation by being imagined as presented to a point of view within that situation, and hence as being experienced as to the left from that point of view. In this way, an experience-relative aspect of a visualised scene, how it and its elements are oriented, is imagined through imagining an experience with the appropriate property'.[18]

When Martin presses the points quoted in the last paragraph, it is in the course of presenting a subtle explanatory argument for the conclusion that one who performs a visualizing thereby imagines a visual sensation from the inside. A reading of Martin's argument will be considered below, in Chapter 3. But his remarks also suggest a less subtle non-explanatory argument for thinking that visualizings must always be imaginings of visual sensations, and indeed for the much stronger conclusion that every distinctively sensory representation is subjective.

Consider a distinctively sensory representation. Suppose that the representation shows, say, a table. As we saw earlier in this chapter, the representation's showing of a table must be perspectival. More specifically, let's assume that the representation shows a table because the representation shows things as *looking* a certain way from a perspective. But, it might be claimed, what it is for things to look a certain way from a perspective just is for things to look that way in the course of a sensation that occurs at the perspective.

To recycle some of Martin's words, the idea of things as looking some way from a point of view might be thought to involve the idea that those things are 'presented to a point of view', and hence that they are 'experienced . . . from that point of view'. (How could there be looks without

---

[18] Martin 2002, 410.

lookers?[19]) If that is right, though, our distinctively sensory representation, in showing a table in a perspectival manner by showing things as looking a certain way from a perspective, must portray a sensation in which things look the relevant way. Hence the distinctively sensory representation is subjective, as it represents a visual sensation from the inside.

More generally, suppose that we are given a distinctively sensory representation. Suppose, first, that the representation shows some item, by showing things as standing sensorily some way. Then the representation shows the thing in a perspectival manner. But, it may seem, what it is for things to stand sensorily some way from a perspective just is for there to be a sensation at the perspective in which things stand sensorily that way. If that is right, though, the representation must be showing things as standing sensorily a certain way in the course of a sensation; it must be portraying a sensation. Hence the representation must be subjective.

Suppose instead, second, that the representation *does not* show any object. (Some sensory mental images of bodily sensations, like stomach aches, might be regarded as fitting that description.) As the representation is distinctively sensory, it shows things as standing sensorily certain ways. But what is left for the representation to do, in showing things as standing sensorily those ways, other than for it to characterize one or more sensations from the inside? The representation must therefore again portray a sensation and must consequently again be subjective.

Either way, though, our distinctively sensory representation is subjective. We thus see, it may be urged, that all distinctively sensory representations—both those which show things and those which do not—are subjective.

<hr>

[19] Currie reports that Walton, in conversation, presented him with an argument which moved directly from the perspectival nature of 'perceptual imagining' to the conclusion that perceptual imaginings are imaginings of sensations (Currie 1995, 188). Currie's response to the argument is to cite examples featuring beliefs as demonstrating—what will be fully borne out below but within the context of a treatment of distinctively sensory representations—that the content of an attitude may be perspectival even though the attitude's content does not refer to some sensory state as being instantiated by the possessor of the attitude (see Currie 1995, 188–9). Moran suggests, too, that 'it is a *formal* property of any such visual representation as an image or a picture that what is shown must be shown from some point of view or other, just as it is a formal property of anything that is thought or conceived of that it is conceived *by someone*. But as with Berkeley's tree in the quad, it doesn't follow that it is part of the content of what is imagined or perceived that it is something imagined or perceived by anyone' (Moran 1994, 92). (Many thanks to an anonymous referee for making me aware of Moran's paper.)

To reflect the visual character of the initial example that prompted the foregoing argument, let's call it the *No Lookerless Looks* argument. The argument has, to my nose, the whiff of sophistry. But the process of thinking about how to respond to it will supply the materials that are needed for explaining how there can be different modes of showing things as standing sensorily certain ways. And the latter modal distinction leads in turn, I will eventually argue, to an explanation of how both objective and subjective distinctively sensory representations are possible.

A line of response

A central assumption of the No Lookerless Looks argument is that what it is for things to stand sensorily some way from a perspective is for the perspective to be the locus of a sensation in which things stand sensorily that way. That assumption may seem pretty anodyne. How could a way for things to stand sensorily be bound to a perspective other than through the occurrence at the perspective of a sensation in which things stand sensorily that way?

That is a good question. But we do seem to be prepared to allow that things may stand sensorily some way from a perspective without the perspective's containing any sensation in which things stand sensorily the relevant way. So, consider a nearby but unoccupied viewpoint *rightwards-perspective* on your right. The chances are that you have a pretty good idea about what things look like from there. And, on the face of it, what you know about is simply a property of *rightwards-perspective*.

Your knowledge of how things look from *rightwards-perspective* may well be based upon thinking about what would be seen by you if you were to occupy *rightwards-perspective*, of course. But that does not mean that your knowledge of how things look from *rightwards-perspective* merely amounts to knowledge of how things would look to you from *rightwards-perspective*. Someone might assess an elephant's actual size by thinking about what the elephant would look like standing next to a bus. Yet the resulting beliefs about the elephant's size would not therefore amount to beliefs about what the elephant would look like standing next to a bus.

Indeed, you might know that things would look a certain way to you if you were to occupy *rightwards-perspective*, while knowing that the relevant way for things to look is not actually how things look from there. For you might know that, if you were to occupy *rightwards-perspective*, your visual system would stop working properly in a predictable way.

Let *Your View* be the type of all and only those visual sensations which are, from the inside, just like the ones which you are now having. Visual sensations of the type *Your View*—*Your View*-sensations—probably do not capture how things look from the perspective *rightwards-perspective* considered in the previous paragraphs. But that fact does not follow merely from the assumption that there is nobody at *rightwards-perspective*; nor does it follow merely from the fact that you would not have a *Your View*-sensation if you were to occupy that perspective.

Instead, *Your View*-sensations do not capture how things look from *rightwards-perspective* because they do not capture what things are like around there. If somebody somewhere is having visual sensations which *do* capture what things are like around *rightwards-perspective*, that person *is* enjoying visual sensations of a type which capture how things look from there.

The idea that things may stand sensorily a certain way from an unoccupied perspective therefore is not at loggerheads with our ordinary ways of thinking. But it needs developing in detail. In particular, what could it mean to say that the sensations of some type capture how things stand sensorily from a perspective because they capture 'what things are like' around there? The following chapter will supply a detailed answer to that question, and thus also to the question how it is that a type of sensations may be bound to a perspective even though the perspective is not occupied by a subject who is having a sensation of the relevant kind.

The resulting ideas will block the No Lookerless Looks argument. But they will also furnish a range of concepts that will be important to the theory of distinctively sensory content articulated in Chapter 3. For the resulting theory of distinctively sensory content will use some ideas developed in the next chapter to refine a thought that surfaced earlier in this one: the thought that there are two modes of showing things as standing sensorily certain ways. In particular, the theory will distinguish between showing things as standing sensorily a certain way 'in the course of a sensation' and showing things as standing sensorily a certain way 'from a perspective'.

2

Matters of Perspective

At the close of the previous chapter, I noted that Chapter 3's theory of distinctively sensory content would divide distinctively sensory representations into two families: first, those which show things as standing sensorily certain ways in the course of sensations; and, second, those which show things as standing sensorily certain ways from perspectives.

Any decent account of either of those two families of representations will need to build upon suitable ideas concerning 'ways for things to stand sensorily'. According to the theory to be developed in Chapter 3, the ways that distinctively sensory representations show things as standing sensorily are types of sensations.[1] This chapter accordingly develops some useful ideas relating to the latter.

It seems clear, too, that any decent account of what it is for a representation to show things as standing sensorily a certain way from a perspective will need to say something about just what it is for things actually to stand sensorily some way from a perspective. A main aim of the current chapter is to meet that demand. It will also develop some ideas that Chapter 3 will eventually bring to bear upon the distinction between subjective and objective distinctively sensory representations. To start things off, though, some preparatory discussion of sensory appearances—for they have been lurking in the background for a while and they will

---

[1] As a number of people have commented to me, there are different usages of phrases like 'the way that things look'; and, on some of those usages, 'ways for things to stand sensorily' are not to be identified with types of sensations. (Talk of 'the way that the table looks' may be used merely to pick out properties that the relevant table appears to possess, for example, like shininess and woodenness.) But our talk of ways that things stand sensorily sometimes does just make reference to types of sensations: I may talk about 'the way that things look' to someone who is suffering a total hallucination, for example, thereby just singling out a type of visual sensations that the person is currently having; or I may say that 'things feel a certain way' in my throat, thereby just identifying the kind of sensations that I am having in my throat.

play a crucial role in this chapter's account of what it is for things to stand sensorily some way from a perspective.

An explanatory distinction

We often distinguish between what literally seems to us to be the case, on account of the sensory experiences which we happen to have, and what we judge to be the case on the basis of how things seem sensorily to us to be. That distinction gestures at a way of explaining the beliefs which ensue from many of our sensations: we are, in the course of sensory episodes, presented with certain putative facts; and, trusting that those putative facts are indeed the case, we judge that appropriate facts must obtain.

According to that explanatory model, our sensations often are not neutral with regard to what the world is like, as they involve presentations of things as being the case. We may then acquiesce in those sensory 'presentations-as-true'[2] and let them guide our subsequent thoughts. But the subsequent thoughts are separate from, and partly explained by, the properly sensory presentations-as-true.

The previous explanatory model is fundamental to our ordinary conception of our minds' lives. And it can hardly be dismissed as mere quackery. For the model's distinction between properly sensory presentations-as-true—sensory appearances—and subsequent judgements is often marked within the phenomenology of our sensory episodes themselves.

Encounters with known examples of sensory illusions supply some of the most striking illustrations of that last point. Consider, for example, Figure 2.1. The lower of the two horizontal lines in that picture looks to

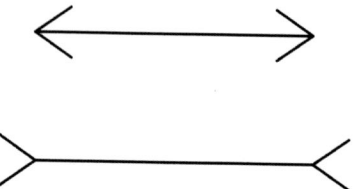

Figure 2.1. The Müller-Lyer illusion

---

[2] This locution is employed in Burge 1993.

be longer than the upper one, although the lines are in fact the same length. Even when we know that the lines are the same length, however, the lengths of the lines still look to us to be different. The visual sensations thus continue to involve sensory appearances which we know better than to trust.[3]

A further range of compelling and obviously relevant examples rely upon cases in which our acquisition of relatively recondite knowledge affects how we respond to what we seem to see. I may on some occasion seem to see a piece of machinery which I cannot identify, for instance, later learning that it was a pillar drill. Suppose that I had been aware, at the earlier time, of what pillar drills look like. Then things might still have looked to be just the same to me—I could have enjoyed the same visual appearances—although my interpretation of what I seemed to see would have been shaped by my awareness of what pillar drills look like. (This is not to claim, of course, that the ways that things look to us cannot ever be affected by our conceptual capacities.)

The rest of this book will take for granted the commonsensical ideas just sketched. It will assume that many of our sensory episodes involve sensory appearances; where our trust in such appearances may, for example, combine with things which we already believe, to lead us to ascribe further significance to the sensations which we have. But the further assumptions about sensory appearances which are employed in the book's theory of distinctively sensory content itself are fairly minimal. In particular, and as noted in the Introduction, the theory will posit certain links between the contents of sensory appearances and distinctively sensory contents, without committing itself to very much at all about the nature of the former.

---

[3] This has been denied; see, for example, Brewer 2006 and Travis 2004 for alternative accounts of what is involved in supposed examples of visual illusions. While the ideas about distinctively sensory contents developed later in this book will rely upon the notion of a sensory appearance, it is worth noting that they do not rely upon the specific sorts of claims about sensory appearances made in the text in relation to Figure 2.1 and other standard examples of sensory illusions; in particular, the later ideas are totally independent of the view that there can be sensations which involve *inaccurate* sensory appearances. Analogous points apply to the next illustrative example provided in the text.

Force and content

Heck remarks that sensory appearances and beliefs are alike in that they 'both . . . have assertoric force'.[4] His statement acknowledges some significant aspects of sensory appearances. It captures, for example, the fact that the sensory appearances which feature in a given sensory episode are like assertions, in that they may be assessed either positively or negatively, depending upon whether they correspond to how things really are. It also reflects how natural it is to factor sensory appearances into two components: force and content.

Consider someone's assertion that $2 + 2 = 5$. That assertion is misplaced, as $2 + 2 \neq 5$. But now compare the assertion to someone's supposition, merely for the sake of argument, that $2 + 2 = 5$. That supposition is not misplaced simply because $2 + 2 \neq 5$. Yet both the supposition and the assertion revolve around the claim that $2 + 2 = 5$. Why do we negatively assess the assertion but not the supposition?

The answer is clear. The assertion amounts to a presentation-as-true of the claim that $2 + 2 = 5$. Hence it is undermined by the fact that $2 + 2 \neq 5$. By contrast, the supposition does not involve the presentation-as-true of the claim that $2 + 2 = 5$. It consequently is not made problematic by the fact that $2 + 2 \neq 5$. While the supposition and the assertion relate to a single content, then, their *forces*—roughly, what they do with their common content—are different.

Sensory appearances have the same sort of force as assertions. For they too amount to presentations-as-true. They are therefore also answerable to how the world is: if the world is not, around me, as my sensory appearances present things as being, the sensory appearances are wrong.[5]

---

[4] Heck 2000, 508. For similar claims by other recent writers, see, for example, Pendlebury 1986, 95; Harman 1990, 34; Yablo 1993, 5; Smith 2001, 308–9; Martin 2002, 386–92; Burge 2003, 542; Peacocke 2004, 99.

[5] Those points are not meant to involve a commitment to a relatively contentious form of representationalism concerning perception. The thought is merely that sensations are sometimes associated with phenomenologically salient accuracy conditions; that is, with phenomenologically salient conditions which the world around the subject must meet if the sensations are to count as being genuine perceptions. The contents which are 'presented as true' in the course of the sensory appearances that figure in some sensation then amount to the phenomenologically salient accuracy conditions with which the sensation is associated. The precise range of philosophical approaches to perception that are consistent with those ideas is a matter for philosophical debate; but see Siegel 2010 for an argument to the effect that any decent

Now, consider the type of visual sensations *Your View* that encompasses just those possible visual sensations that are, from the inside, exactly like those which you are now having. To employ a useful locution of a type that I will use a lot hereafter when singling out the contents of sensory appearances, let's say that it looks to you as though things are *thus*. Then it will look as though things are precisely *thus* to anyone who has a *Your View*-sensation. The way for things to look *Your View* is therefore associated with a range of sensory appearances whose overall content is *things being thus*.

More generally, suppose that every possible sensation of a particular type involves its seeming to the sensation's subject that things are certain specific ways. Suppose, that is, that there are certain ways for things to be which meet the following condition: any possible sensation of the relevant type is a sensation in which things seem to the sensation's subject to be those ways. Then the sensation-type's *appearance-content* amounts to 'things being those ways'. That is, the type's appearance-content embodies exactly the shared ways that things must seem to be to those who have sensations of the relevant type; we saw in the previous paragraph, for instance, that the appearance-content of *Your View* is *things being thus*.

Perspectives

Imagine that someone other than you has a *Your View*-sensation on some occasion. The precise conditions under which the visual appearances forming part of that other person's visual sensations are right or wrong— under which they are or are not *veridical*—are different from the conditions under which the visual appearances which formed part of your own *Your View*-sensation counted as veridical. While the sensory appearances which the other person is having will be veridical just in case things are, around her, *thus*, things do need to be *thus* around her; whereas the veridicality of your visual appearances required that things should be *thus* around you.

The contents of the visual appearances associated with *Your View* therefore do not determine on their own the veridicality-conditions belonging to the sensory appearances that accompany any particular

philosophical approach to perception—including standard forms of 'naive realism'—will allow for sensations that have accuracy conditions in the previous sense.

possible *Your View*-sensation. While the veridicality-conditions belonging to the sensory appearances accompanying a particular possible *Your View*-sensation involve things being *thus* somewhere, the specific circumstances in which things must be *thus* need also to be fixed. And, to fix the identity of those circumstances, suitable aspects of the context containing the relevant possible *Your View*-sensation need to be taken into account.

Suppose that the members of one of those groups of further contextual features are bundled together—as an ordered *n*-tuple, say, in the logicians' style. Then it makes sense to consider whether things are *thus* relative to the bundle. The bundle is therefore a *perspective*. Indeed, the bundle is a 'visual' perspective, as it makes sense to consider whether the appearance-content of some way for things to look is true or false relative to the bundle.[6] More particularly, however, whether or not things are *thus* relative to the relevant bundle of contextual features determines whether the sensory appearances that form part of a certain sensation are in fact veridical. The relevant sensation therefore *occurs* at the perspective; and the perspective is therefore *occupied*.[7]

I shall now explore in more detail the natures of the perspectives at which auditory and visual sensations occur. This is partly to fill out the very schematic and abstract ideas just presented. But it will also provide me with some ideas relating specifically to vision and hearing which will be useful at various later points.

It is worth emphasizing, in passing, the inherent generality of the notion of a sensory perspective. Sensory perspectives are merely groups of contextual factors relative to which the appearance-contents of ways for things to stand sensorily are true or false. While the specific features soon to be ascribed to visual and auditory perspectives may or may not also be

---

[6] Note that this talk of 'truth' should not be taken as involving a commitment to the idea that the contents of sensory appearances are propositional and hence conceptual; see Chapter 4 for more discussion of the distinction between conceptual and non-conceptual contents. If the reader is uncomfortable with talking about the 'truth' of the contents of sensory appearances—for example, on account of wishing to preserve the common view that propositions are the primary bearers of truth and falsity (as, for example, Burge 2010, 39 and 280)—he or she is welcome mentally to substitute all of this book's talk of the perspectival truth and falsity of the contents of sensory appearances with, say, talk of their perspectival 'correctness' and 'incorrectness'.

[7] To simplify things, I have bound specific perspectives to particular possible worlds in what follows. So, for example, this world is the only possible world which contains the very perspectives at which your current visual sensations are occurring.

possessed by the perspectives that are associated with other forms of sensation, there is nothing essentially visual or auditory in the concept of a sensory perspective itself. More generally, the theory of distinctively sensory content presented in Chapter 3 contains nothing that is essentially bound just to seeing and hearing, even though—with our sensory powers being as they are—visual and auditory cases will provide me with many of the most compelling illustrations of aspects of distinctively sensory content.

Occupied auditory and visual perspectives

What are the components of the perspectives at which, say, *Your View*-sensations occur? The specific conditions under which the visual appearances accompanying a particular *Your View*-sensation count as veridical obviously depend upon the spatiotemporal location of the sensing subject. Those specific conditions also derive from orientational facts. For a given *Your View*-sensation makes it look to the subject that various sorts of things are situated in various interrelated directions, directions which we might roughly but aptly single out using orientational language like 'directly-forwards', 'just-left-of-directly-forwards-and-up-a-bit', and so on.

We can capture the contribution made by a subject's spatiotemporal location to determining the precise conditions under which some particular possible *Your View*-appearances count as veridical by taking a cue from Peacocke's discussion of the 'representational content of experience'.[8] For we may assume that the perspective at which the sensation occurs includes an *origin*: a place in a possible world at a time. And we can capture the contribution of orientational factors to fixing those veridicality-conditions by assuming that the perspective also includes a suitable system of *labelled axes*, where the relevant axes indicate directions around the perspective's origin.

Consider the location of a subject of a possible *Your View*-sensation. We can label all sorts of directions running off from the subject's position using orientational labels like 'directly-forwards', 'straight-upwards', and the rest. But many of the resulting groups of labelled axes which relate to our chosen subject's position will not fix the veridicality-conditions of the

---

[8] Peacocke 1992, 61.

appearances which the subject has enjoyed. If it looks to our subject as though something of a certain sort is directly-forwards, for instance, those appearances will be veridical only if something suitable is located in one of the directions that runs away from his location: the direction that is 'presented to him' as directly-forwards by his *Your View*-sensation.

The particular group of labelled axes included in the perspective at which our subject's *Your View*-sensation occurs is the one which labels as 'directly-forwards' the direction which is presented to him as directly-forwards by his *Your View*-sensation, which labels as 'just-to-the-left-of-directly-forwards' the direction which is presented to him as just-to-the-left-of-directly-forwards by his *Your View*-sensation, and so on. But nothing in the preceding discussion had anything particular to do with the idiosyncratic nature of *Your View*. It is accordingly natural to think that each occupied visual perspective will contain an origin and a suitable system of labelled axes.

What will figure in occupied auditory perspectives? As in the visual case, the specific conditions under which some auditory appearances count as veridical depend upon the spatial location of the sensing subject. Occupied auditory perspectives will therefore also need to include origins that are tagged to particular places.

A potential complication arises at this point. I earlier identified the origins of the perspectives at which *Your View*-sensations occur with places in possible worlds at particular times. I thus assumed that *Your View*-sensations are momentary in nature. But that may be wrong: some philosophers have argued that it is a mistake to regard extended visual episodes as constituted by sequences of momentary snapshot-like visual sensations.[9] Whether or not vision is like that, however, I myself find it fairly natural to hold that there are no momentary snapshot-like auditory sensations. It may be, then, that the origins of the perspectives at which auditory (and indeed visual) sensations occur ought not to be identified with places in possible worlds at single times.

But that is not a problem. If auditory episodes, for instance, are not composed of momentary snapshot-like auditory sensations then we should simply identify the origins of the perspectives in which auditory sensations occur with particular places in possible worlds during *intervals* of time. Note too that, while the last suggestion reflects the appealing thought that

---

[9] See, for example, O'Shaughnessy 2000, 47–9; and Phillips 2010.

shifts in a listener's spatial position result in shifts in the auditory perspectives that the listener occupies, one could in principle further liberalize the demands upon auditory perspectives. One could, say, allow for perspectives whose origins involve a multiplicity of different places during temporal intervals. The availability of all these options reflects the inherent generality of the notion of a sensory perspective.

Do occupied auditory perspectives need also to incorporate suitable systems of labelled axes? It seems clear that they ought sometimes to include them. So, the auditory appearances which I am currently enjoying exhibit an auditorily defined directional structure that is broadly analogous to the visually defined directional structure which is manifested by my current visual sensations. Some of the various sounds that I am now hearing sound to me to be coming from the right, for example, while others sound to me to be coming from behind. The perspectives at which my current auditory sensations are occurring should therefore be taken to include appropriate systems of labelled axes.

It is not wholly clear that auditory appearances are always perspectivally directional in broadly the same sort of way as visual appearances, however. (Responses to my own claims to the contrary in earlier drafts of this book have brought that point home to me.) Yet that is not a difficulty. For suppose that there can be auditory sensations whose accompanying auditory appearances are not perspectivally directional. Then, while the auditory perspectives at which those sensations occur should certainly be taken to include origins, the sensations' lack of perspectival directionality may be reflected simply by the *absence* of labelled axes in those occupied perspectives. I have sometimes spoken below as though occupied auditory perspectives need always to include systems of labelled axes, however, just to avoid further clutter.

Do the perspectives at which auditory and visual sensations occur need to include more than origins and suitable systems of labelled axes? The answer to that question will depend upon the resolution of certain very general questions about the nature of the contents of auditory and visual appearances, questions which I will not attempt to answer in this book.

Suppose, for instance, that the appearances involved in visual sensations of type T make it seem to the subject that, very roughly, '*that* thing just in front is red'. Then there will be, in a sense, a single way that things seem to be to the possible subjects of T-sensations. Yet the item which counts as 'that' thing in relation to one T-sensation may be distinct from the item which counts as 'that' thing in relation to another *T*-sensation. In that case, though, different veridicality-conditions will be associated with the appearances that are enjoyed by the subjects of the relevant distinct possible *T*-sensations.

The perspective at which some possible *T*-sensation occurs is the bundle of contextual features which fix the veridicality-conditions for the sensory appearances accompanying the relevant sensation. Given our initial assumptions, then, the perspectives at which *T*-sensations occur will need to include factors which settle what counts as 'that' thing in relation to the specific *T*-sensation at issue. Those potential complications will be irrelevant to the later parts of this book, however. I will therefore keep things simple, by speaking as though occupied auditory and visual perspectives do not need to incorporate any more than origins and appropriate systems of labelled axes.

The next section discusses empty sensory perspectives: bundles of contextual features relative to which the contents of sensory appearances may be true or false, even though no sensations occur at the relevant perspectives. The resulting discussion will set things up for the end of the chapter, which argues that—contrary to what was assumed in the No Lookerless Looks argument—things may stand sensorily certain ways from empty perspectives.

Empty perspectives

Take some perspective *p* at which a *Your View*-sensation occurs. Let's assume for the sake of definiteness that *p* consists entirely of an origin *o*—your whereabouts when you had your own earlier *Your View*-sensation—and the group of labelled axes *L*, which captures the directions around *o* as they were earlier presented to you by your past *Your View*-sensation.

Now consider a related bundle of contextual features *p**: *p** consists of the same origin *o* but a different group *L** of labelled axes around *o*. More specifically, *L** flips all of the directions around *o* as defined by *L*; that is, *L** labels the direction which is opposite to *L*'s *directly-forwards* direction as 'directly-forwards', *L** labels the direction which is opposite to *L*'s *just-left-of-directly-forwards-and-up-a-bit* direction as 'just-left-of-directly-forwards-and-up-a-bit', and so on.

The appearances involved in your earlier *Your View*-sensation were veridical just in case the world was laid out suitably around *o*. In particular, it seemed to you that things were *thus*; and the appearances which you enjoyed were veridical just in case things were *thus* around *o*, relative to the directions around *o* defined by *L*. Let's suppose that the appearances which you enjoyed in the course of your *Your View*-sensation were veridical. But let's also assume that how things then were behind you did not amount to a flipped-over version of the way that things then looked to you to be. Things therefore were not *thus* around *o*, relative to the directions around *o* defined by *L**.

While things were not *thus* relative to *o* and *L**—that is, relative to the perspective *p**—it obviously made perfect sense to consider whether or not things were *thus* relative to *p**. And that is simply because *p** contained suitable counterparts of the components of your earlier perspective *p*. So, while the bundle of contextual features *p** is not a perspective at which some visual sensation actually occurred, it is nonetheless a visual perspective: it is an empty one.

Empty visual and auditory perspectives seem to be unproblematic. When things look or sound a certain way to us, we may surely latch onto places that are not occupied by sensing subjects, and consider, in relation to various ways of setting up directions around those places, whether things are around there as they look or sound to us to be. (Similarly, we will see at the very end of this chapter that empty tactile perspectives seem to be unproblematic.) Yet perhaps those intuitive thoughts merely reflect our failure to think in enough detail about the perspectives at which visual and auditory sensations occur. In particular, let's reconsider the labels which are attached to the directions found in the groups of labelled axes included within visual and auditory perspectives.

Those labels are meant to reflect the ways in which orientational facts are apparently presented to us 'in the phenomenology of [auditory and visual] experience itself'.[10] Evans asks, though, 'how we might specify the spatial information which we imagine [an auditory] perception to embody'. His answer is that '[t]he subject hears the sound as coming from such-and-such a position', where the relevant position needs to be specified 'in *egocentric* terms (he hears the sound as up, or down, to the right or to the left, in front or behind)'. And, he says, '[t]hese terms specify the position of the sound in relation to the observer's own body; and they derive their meaning in part from their complicated connections with the subject's *actions*'.[11]

Suppose that Evans is right, though, and that his points extend to vision. Suppose, that is, that the orientational structures of visual and auditory appearances arise from its seeming to us that visible things and sounds stand in certain sorts of action-involving relationships to our bodies. Then—depending upon the precise nature of the relevant action-involving relationships—the labels which feature in the groups of labelled axes included in auditory and visual perspectives may have to be understood as singling out directions in terms of their action-involving relationships to the bodies of sensing subjects. But the very labels featuring in the groups of labelled axes would then presuppose that the perspectives are occupied.

On the face of it, however, it is bizarre to think that auditory and visual directions derive from apparent action-involving relationships between sights, sounds, and our conscious selves. Auditory and visual appearances present the world as oriented in relation to an implicitly defined spatial centre, for sure. But they do not seem also to insist on the presence of a certain sort of conscious thing at the relevant centre, one whose presence there is what settles questions about the orientational relationships holding among what is apparently seen or heard.

Evans observes, though, that:

---

[11]   That quotation and the preceding ones from Evans are from Evans 1982, 155; see also, for example, Noë 2004, 87–8, for parallel claims about forms of sensory experience more generally. Evans cites, on p. 156, a passage from Taylor which says that '[o]ur perceptual field has an orientational structure, a foreground and a background, an up and down . . . What is [the up–down directionality] based on? Up and down are not simply related to my body—up is not just where my head is and down where my feet are. For I can be lying down, or bending over, or upside down; and in all these cases "up" in my field is not the direction of my head . . . Rather, up and down are related to how one would move and act in the field' (Taylor 1978–9, 154). (While Evans, Taylor, and Noë take the spatial content of auditory appearances to be somehow bound to possibilities of movement, an alternative and more radical view—one whose falsity is just assumed in the text for introspective reasons—would have it that, in hearing, we do not enjoy sensory appearances which have spatial contents at all; rather, 'sounds have no position in space . . . we associate them with movements, and in that way they serve the purpose of warning us of those movements, of appearing to make them necessary and natural' (Proust [1920] 1989, 72).)

[w]hen we hear a sound as coming from a certain direction, we do not have to *think* or *calculate* which way to turn our heads (say) in order to look for the source of the sound. If we did have to do so, then it ought to be possible for two people to hear a sound as coming from the same direction . . . and yet to be disposed to do quite different things in reacting to the sound, because of differences in their calculations. Since this does not appear to make sense, we must say that having spatially significant perceptual information consists at least partly in being disposed to do various things.[12]

Evans is evidently right to claim that the orientational information with which we are provided by our auditory sensations is typically immediately available for use in guiding behaviour. But the mere fact that the relevant information is straight away available for behavioural uptake does not nearly imply that the information's content somehow relates to our behavioural dispositions. The observed immediacy can be explained, for instance, merely by supposing that our brains somehow automatically and unconsciously map directions as they are presented to us in the course of auditory sensations onto directions as they are presented to us by our bodily senses.[13]

How about the second part of Evans's comments, his claim that it is just senseless to suppose that two people might hear a sound as coming from a single direction and yet be disposed to behave differently in reacting to the sound?

That seems to be false. There is nothing nonsensical about the idea that two subjects might have, say, visual appearances with the same orientational structures even though their dispositions to react to what they seem to see vary radically. In fact, there seem actually to be subjects who enjoy normal visual and auditory appearances yet whose behavioural dispositions in relation to those appearances are radically different from those which we possess. People who suffer from optic 'ataxia', for example, show a 'marked incoordination, slowness and inaccuracy of visually-elicited

---

[12] Evans 1982, 155. Peacocke states, too, that '[i]n supplying a subject with information about the location of things relative to bodily axes, perception supplies that nonconceptual information in a form immediately usable if the subject wants to move his body or some limb toward, from, or in some other spatial relation to what he perceives' (Peacocke 1992, 93).

[13] Peacocke himself probably sees the need for this sort of mapping in at least some cases; he comments that 'in the specification of the representational content of some human experiences, one would need to consider several . . . systems of origins and axes, and to specify the spatial relations of these systems to one another' (1992, 63).

hand movements', while otherwise evincing no 'significant motor, pro-prioceptive, visual field or visual space perception disturbances'. Analogous points apply to those who are afflicted by auditory ataxia.[14]

The issues raised here deserve further discussion. But it would take me too far afield from my main concerns to provide a more extended treatment of them. It should be noted, though, that the views concerning empty perspectives and labelled axes that I have just endorsed are wholly detachable from the theory of distinctively sensory content developed in the next chapter. Rather, they are merely some premises which I will call upon: first, in replying to the No Lookerless Looks argument presented in Chapter 1; and, second, in Chapter 3's attempt to explain how objective distinctively sensory representations are possible.

'From perspectives'

Consider a viewpoint which is near to you. What do things look like from there? As noted towards the end of the previous chapter, you may answer that question by identifying a way for things to look which captures what things are like around the relevant perspective. *Your View* probably is not a way that things look from the perspective, for example, because things doubtless are not *thus* around the perspective. But perhaps you can produce a visual mental image which shows things as looking like *that*, where things are like *that* around the relevant perspective. If so, the way that your visual mental image shows things as looking is a way that things look from the perspective.

More generally, consider a way for things to stand sensorily T. Suppose that T's appearance-content is *things being like this*. The contents of the sensory appearances associated with T capture what things are like around perspective p just in case things are like *this* relative to p. But T is a way that things stand sensorily from p just in case the contents of T's associated sensory appearances capture what things are like around p. Hence we have the following:

---

[14] See Perenin and Vighetto 1988, 661, for the passage quoted in the previous sentence. (One of the patients being considered there suffered from auditory as well as optic ataxia ('Apart from Case 6 who showed some degree of "auditory ataxia" . . . ', on the same page).) See Clark 2001 for more discussion of these issues.

(2.A)   A sensation-type T is a way that things stand sensorily from a perspective just in case T's appearance-content is true relative to the perspective.

(The indefinite article in the phrase 'a way that things stand sensorily from a perspective' in (2.A) above is essential; there will generally be many ways that things stand sensorily from a given perspective.)

Principle (2.A) provides a general account of what it is for things to stand sensorily a certain way from a perspective. The following chapter will use this principle to provide an account of what it is for a distinctively sensory representation to show things as standing sensorily a certain way from a perspective. Principle (2.A) will therefore be pivotal to this book's account of one of the two modes of showing things as standing sensorily a certain way.

An argument refuted

To conclude this chapter, let's return to the No Lookerless Looks argument presented in Chapter 1. The crucial part of that argument went as follows. Suppose that a distinctively sensory representation shows something. Then the representation shows what it shows in a perspectival manner. But what it is for things to stand sensorily some way from a perspective just is for the perspective to belong to a sensing subject to whom things stand sensorily that way. The representation must therefore show things as standing sensorily a certain way to a sensing subject. So the representation portrays a sensation.

That argument turns on the assumption that what it is for things to stand sensorily some way from a perspective just is for the perspective to belong to a sensing subject to whom things stand sensorily that way. Yet that assumption may be rejected, given principle (2.A) and various other independently plausible premisses.

In the course of visual sensations, we seem to see all sorts of things. Perhaps some of what we seem to see sometimes relates to mentality. Maybe, for example, it sometimes literally looks to us as though people are happy or sad, rather than merely that the parts of their faces are arranged in certain ways. But there are very many visual sensations in which the diverse putative facts that are thereby presented to us as obtaining have this in common: none of them concerns our own mental lives, nor do any of them concern the mental lives of any other subjects.[15] Similar remarks apply to many other sorts of sensations, including auditory and tactile ones.[16]

Consider the way that things look to you right now. That is, consider the type *Your Newest View* covering exactly those possible sensations which are subjectively indiscernible from your own current visual sensation. I'll assume that the visual appearances that you are currently having are veridical. I'll assume, that is, that *Your Newest View*'s appearance-content—*things being such-and-such*, let's say—is true relative to your own viewpoint. Finally, I take it that whether things are *such-and-such* relative to a given perspective has nothing to do with any facts about what things are like within the mental lives of any subjects.

There could surely be an empty but otherwise indiscernible copy of your current perspective. Consider, for instance, a possible situation that is just like your own, except that it contains a zombified version of you. *Your Newest View*'s appearance-content would be true relative to that empty perspective. For, apart from the fact that the counterpart perspective is empty, things are around there just as they are around you. And the counterpart's emptiness—the fact that no sensations occur at the perspective—is totally irrelevant to whether things are *such-and-such* in relation to it, because *Your Newest View*'s appearance-content is silent about mental matters. So things will be *such-and-such* in relation to the counterpart perspective, just as they are *such-and-such* around you.

The appearance-content of *Your Newest View* could therefore be true relative to an empty perspective. But (2.A) tells us that *Your Newest View* is a way that things look from a perspective just in case the sensation-type's appearance-content is true relative to the perspective. So *Your Newest View*

---

[15] This claim is more contentious than it may sound. Quite apart from a well-known view endorsed by Searle and noted in a footnote in the previous chapter, some philosophers have argued that our visual sensations, when they present things to us as being external, thereby present apparently seen items as being independent of those very sensations. For a recent argument along those lines, see Siegel 2006, who claims that, in presenting apparently viewed items as external (see in particular p. 374 of Siegel's paper), the contents of visual appearances make references to how things would look to us if we were to change our positions in relevant ways. I think that these arguments are mistaken because they rely upon incorrect accounts of the apparent externality that is involved in visual appearances; see this book's conclusion for more on all this. Anyway, the points being introduced in the text certainly are not essential to the theory of distinctively sensory content articulated in the next chapter, although I suspect that they would be widely endorsed.

[16] See Armstrong 1962, 31–2, for more discussion of the tactile case.

could be a way that things look from an empty perspective. Things may therefore stand sensorily a certain way from a perspective even though there is nobody at the perspective to whom things stand sensorily that way. The No Lookerless Looks argument is therefore unsound.

Indeed, it is hardly surprising that things can look or sound certain ways from empty perspectives. Visual and auditory sensations often purport merely to tell us about what our physical environments are like; they often do not purport to tell us about what, in mental terms, things are like for us or for anyone else. So why wouldn't the specifications of our surroundings which are given by the visual or auditory sensations of some kind sometimes characterize what things are like around empty perspectives?

What holds there for visual and auditory sensations may hold for sensations of other kinds as well. Put your feet on the floor. The resulting tactile sensations feature certain sensory appearances of contact and pressure, ones that are veridical just in case things are in fact appropriate ways relative to certain bodily regions.[17] Let's assume that the appearances are veridical. Furthermore, I take it that the tactile appearances are silent about mental matters.

Consider an unconscious copy of you, a copy whose surroundings are also an exact copy of your own. The contents of the tactile appearances which you are having capture what things are like relative to those regions of the copy's body which correspond to the relevant regions of your own body. But the corresponding regions of the copy's body are empty perspectives;[18] and the appearance-contents of the ways that your feet

---

[17] The task of providing a satisfactory account of the nature of tactile perspectives is actually rather more difficult than suggested by the simple talk of 'bodily regions' in the text. But it seems clear that, whatever exactly tactile perspectives amount to, the points made in the following paragraph will still go through.

[18] An empty tactile perspective is a bundle of contextual features relative to which it makes sense to consider whether the contents of some tactile appearances obtain, but which does not determine the veridicality-conditions for the sensory appearances accompanying any specific possible sensation. A tactile perspective may thus be 'empty' even though its origin is not a wholly vacant spatiotemporal location. I think that the appearance-contents of visual and auditory sensation-types can be true relative to perspectives whose origins feature patches of empty space. But the appearance-contents of tactile sensation-types are not like this, because tactile appearances purport to present us with instances of *contact* (see, for instance, Armstrong 1962, 11).

just felt to you by touch are true relative to those empty perspectives. Principle (2.A)'s general account of what it is for things to stand sensorily some way from a perspective then tells us that there can be empty perspectives from which things feel the ways that things felt to you in the course of your recent foot-centred tactile sensations.

3

A Theory of Distinctively Sensory Content

The current chapter presents this book's theory of distinctively sensory content: it explains how the members of the class of representations which show things as standing sensorliy certain ways are united in possessing contents of a special sort.

The chapter's first two sections address some pressing questions. What is it for a representation to 'show' things as, say, looking some way? And how does a certain representation that shows things as looking some way manage thereby also to 'show' worldly items like tables and chairs? I hold that the contents of distinctively sensory representations single out ways for things to stand sensorily—types of sensations—in a special manner. The involvement of those special modes of presentation is what accounts for the fact that distinctively sensory representations may perform the two sorts of showings cited in the previous two questions.

Distinctively sensory representations are alike in possessing contents which single out ways for things to stand sensorily in a distinctive fashion. But the chapter also argues, following up a suggestion first made in Chapter 1, that there are two modes of showing how things stand sensorily. There is, first, showing things as standing sensorily some way in the course of a sensation. And there is, second, showing things as standing sensorily some way from a perspective.

A theoretical account of the two different sorts of distinctively sensory contents which answer to those two modes of showing how things stand sensorily is provided below. The account of what it is to show things as standing sensorily some way in the course of a sensation will start from an obvious thought about what it is for things actually to stand sensorily some way in the course of a sensation. And the account of what it is to show things as standing sensorily a certain way from a perspective will call heavily upon the previous chapter's ideas concerning what it is for things actually to stand sensorily some way from a perspective.

The chapter's remaining sections use its theory of distinctively sensory content for some relatively abstract explanatory purposes. In particular, the theory is used to explain all of the characteristic constraints that were identified in Chapter 1 as affecting distinctively sensory representations, along with an open-ended array of similar constraints. The theory is also combined with some additional but independently plausible premises, to provide an explanation of how there can be both subjective and objective distinctively sensory representations. The resulting combination of views will also briefly be related to a notable argument concerning visualization, at the chapter's close.

Subjective informativeness

Suppose that you view a photograph, thereby grasping that the photo shows things as looking a certain way. What do you appreciate when you grasp that the photo shows things as looking the relevant way?

Consider possible worlds semantics, perhaps the currently dominant theoretical approach to the contents of linguistic representations. When we understand a declarative sentence like 'Sheffield is larger than Shiptonthorpe', we appreciate the way that the sentence states that things stand. Possible worlds semanticists treat the information which we thereby acquire as amounting to a distinction between two families of possible worlds. There are, first, the possible worlds in which Sheffield is larger than Shiptonthorpe. And there are, second, the possible worlds in which Sheffield is not larger than Shiptonthorpe.

We may, likewise, treat your appreciation of a way that a photo shows things as looking as amounting to a grasp of the distinction between two families of visual sensations. There are, first, those visual sensations in which things look the way that the photo shows them as looking. And there are, second, those visual sensations in which things do not look that way. More generally, it is pretty natural to identify the ways for things to stand sensorily involved in distinctively sensory contents with types of sensations, as I have done.

Distinctively sensory contents presumably 'involve' types of sensations by somehow singling them out. But there are many different ways in which categories of sensations may be identified. I can, while clenching my toes, single out just those apparent toe-clenchings that feel like *this*; but I can also pick out just those kinaesthetic and tactile sensations that are currently enjoyed by people wearing red socks. I can, too, pick out just those kinaesthetic and tactile sensations in which the subject's arm apparently moves; or just those that are had by subjects who are now standing in the rain.

Suppose again that you view a photograph, thereby grasping that the photo shows things as looking a certain way. Your appreciation of a way that the photo shows things as looking has the potential to lead you to a striking range of further abilities. If your memory is working properly, for example, then you should be able to ascertain in the moments soon after viewing the photo whether things actually look to you the way that you took the photo to show things as looking. Or you may be able to survey some of your visual memories, leading you to realize that things once looked to you the way that you took the photo to show things as looking.

Some ways of singling out types of visual sensations are incapable of underwriting those sorts of capacities. Imagine that you are passed a sealed envelope which contains a photo, for instance. And suppose that you are forbidden to open the envelope, instead just being told that the photo inside captures the way that things looked to me at precisely 9.52 a.m. yesterday. That information alone will not help you to ascertain in the near future whether things actually look to you the way just specified. Nor will it allow you to survey your visual memories to assess whether things once looked to you the relevant way. Why so?

The crucial point is that your mere awareness that the photo captures the way that things looked to me at precisely 9.52 a.m. yesterday does not lead you to appreciate *what it is like* to have a visual sensation in which things look that way. So, suppose you were somehow to learn what it is like to have a sensation in which things look the way that things looked to me at precisely 9.52 a.m. yesterday; perhaps you eventually open the envelope and sneak a look at the photo inside. You should then be able to connect your knowledge about the way that the photo shows things as looking with, say, your own subsequent visual sensations.

The kinds of abilities just considered are ones that always have the potential to arise from understandings of distinctively sensory representations. And, just intuitively, their potential to arise flows from the fact that distinctively sensory representations *show* things as standing sensorily certain ways. To take another example, produce some olfactory mental imagery. You should be able to ascertain whether the way that things actually smell to you now is the way that your olfactory mental image showed things as smelling. And perhaps you realize that the way your olfactory mental image showed things as smelling is a way that things actually once smelled to you.

In showing things as standing sensorily certain ways, then, distinctively sensory representations have the potential to underwrite the sorts of capacities roughly outlined above. But I take it that distinctively sensory representations 'show' things as standing sensorily certain ways because of the distinctive manner in which their contents pick out ways for things to stand sensorily. There must therefore be special links between the ways in which distinctively sensory contents single out types of sensations and facts about what it is like to have sensations of the relevant types. How might those special links arise?

Here is the straightforward answer to that question that is assumed below:

(3.A)   Distinctively sensory contents single out ways for things to stand sensorily in *subjectively informative* ways: they single out types of sensations just in terms of what it is like to have sensations of the relevant kinds.[1] And that is why distinctively sensory representations *show* things as standing sensorily certain ways.

Distinctively sensory contents thus pick out types of sensations in a broadly descriptive manner: they identify ways for things to stand sensorily simply by isolating the subjective characters that are common to all and only the possible sensations of the relevant types. To capture (3.A) with a slogan: *Distinctively sensory showing comes from subjective informativeness.*

The thesis that *distinctively sensory showing*—'showing things as standing sensorily certain ways'—*comes from subjective informativeness* provides the most straightforward explanation of the facts about distinctively sensory

---

[1] The notion of subjective informativeness is evidently bound up with the idea of a subject's appreciation of what it is like for things to stand sensorily a certain way; and that notion (or close relatives of it) have been central to many discussions of physicalism about the mental. (See, for example, Lewis 1988; Nemirow 1990; and Conee 1994.) This book will not assume any particular theoretical approach to the idea of a subject's being aware of what it is like for things to stand sensorily some way. And all of the ways in which that notion is employed below are, I think, ones that would need to be recoverable from any decent account of how the idea works.

representations and potential abilities noted earlier. Your understanding of a photo may lead you to appreciate that the photo shows things as looking a certain way, for instance. You thus identify a way for things to look in terms of what it is like to have a sensation in which things look that way. Your understanding of the photo therefore features a component—your awareness of what it is like to have visual sensations of a certain sort—that can underpin various abilities of the kind outlined previously.

The suggested link between distinctively sensory showing and subjective informativeness has a lot of intuitive appeal. So, produce a gustatory mental image. Consider the way that your image shows things as tasting. What is it for a sensation to be of that type? Surely the answer is just this: things taste the relevant way to a subject precisely if the subject has a gustatory sensation possessing a certain subjective character—one in which things are like *that* for her, as you might put it. The mode of presentation by means of which your gustatory mental image picks out the way that it shows things as tasting thus does seem to be subjectively informative. But the mental image's peculiarly subjective identification of the way that it shows things as standing sensorily—as encompassing exactly those possible gustatory sensations in which things are like *that*—is also what one registers when one states that the mental image 'shows' things as tasting a certain way.

The claim that *distinctively sensory showing comes from subjective informativeness* fits well, too, with the evident contrasts between various sorts of cases. I am able to provide a verbal description of the way that things look to me right now: 'I seem to see a computer screen with a loudspeaker next to it, both of which stand in front of a wall that has lots of pictures by children stuck to it; the computer screen has some letters of the alphabet on it . . .'. Yet I take it that the verbal description does not single out the way that things look to me by identifying the subjective character which is common to just those possible sensations in which things look the relevant way. The description's content therefore lacks the special connection to vision's felt character that makes for distinctively sensory showing. (There is further discussion of the relationships between linguistic representations and distinctively sensory ones in the next chapter.)

The subjective informativeness of distinctively sensory contents is a matter of the modes of presentation under which they single out types of sensations; it is, to use the Fregean terminology, an aspect of their *senses*.[2]

---

[2] Frege [1892a] 1997.

The fact that *distinctively sensory showing comes from subjective informativeness* also constrains the range of types of sensations which can be ways that distinctively sensory representations show things as standing sensorily. For a type of sensations is then fit to figure in a distinctively sensory content only if there is some subjective character which is common to all and only the type's possible instances—only if there is a 'what it's like'-ness which is common to all and only the possible sensations of the relevant kind.

Precisely which groupings of sensations are let through by that last constraint? Is there a subjective character which is shared by, say, all and only the possible gustatory sensations? I do not know the answers to those questions; nor do I need to know their answers for the purposes of this book. There are some cases which I take to be fairly clear-cut, however.

I take it that there is no subjective character which is common to all and only those possible visual sensations in which a subject 'seems to see a table', for instance. While there may be some 'what it's like'-ness which is shared by each possible visual sensation in which someone seems to see a table, the relevant subjective character will surely be so general as to be shared by other visual sensations which are not of that kind. Hence it seems that there is no subjective character which is common to all *and only* those possible visual sensations in which a table—whether small or large, wooden or metal, brown or blue, gate-leg or drop-leaf . . . —is apparently seen.

Scene-showing

We speak of 'showing' in a wide variety of circumstances. Someone may show me a table, for example; I may show someone how to get from Crookes to Ughill; and somebody might show me that my arguments contain flaws. The previous section proposed a theoretical approach to one notable use of 'showing' talk. The resulting ideas concerning distinctively sensory showing—'showing things as standing sensorily certain ways'—were not meant to embody a theory of showing in full generality. But there are some additional uses of 'showing' talk which need further consideration.

Many distinctively sensory representations do not just show things as standing sensorily certain ways. In showing things as looking certain ways, for example, pictures and visual mental images may thereby show scenes containing such things as tables and chairs. Now, it is not evident that distinctively sensory representations always show worldly items by showing things as standing sensorily certain ways: it is not clear that a sensory mental image of an itch does any more than to characterize the felt nature of a sensory episode, for instance. But the showings of items that many distinctively sensory representations do accomplish by means of showing things as standing sensorily certain ways are particularly important to this book.

Those derived showings were central to Chapter 1's identifications of some telling representational constraints applying to distinctively sensory representations, for instance. To take one case, we saw there that distinctively sensory representations that show items like tables and chairs, by showing things as looking certain ways, must always show the relevant items from perspectives. It will sometimes be helpful to have some terminology for explicitly singling out the showings of items that distinctively sensory representations may perform by showing things as standing sensorily certain ways: I shall call them *scene-showings* when special emphasis is needed.

The thesis that *distinctively sensory showing comes from subjective informativeness* has significant consequences for scene-showings. Suppose that a picture shows a chair, by showing things as looking a certain way. The picture 'shows'—rather than just represents—a chair, on account of the fact that the picture presents a chair in an especially visual fashion. That point may be smoothly accommodated by appealing to the principle that *distinctively sensory showing comes from subjective informativeness.*

Our hypothetical picture shows a chair because it shows things as looking a certain way. More fully, the picture shows a chair because, for some way *T* that the picture shows things as looking, part of what it is for things to look that way to a subject is for the person to seem to see a chair. But *distinctively sensory showing comes from subjective informativeness.* The picture's content thus singles out *T* precisely in terms of what it is like to have a sensory episode in which things look that way.

A chair of some sort is therefore being picked out by the picture, through its singling out of *T*, in terms of what it is like to seem to see a chair of the relevant type. The picture thus does indeed present a chair in a peculiarly visual manner. And we record the fact that the picture presents a chair in terms of what it is like to seem to see a chair of the relevant variety by stating that the picture 'shows' a chair.

That example illustrates a significant general point. The nature of the items which are scene-shown by some distinctively sensory representation is determined by the nature of the sensory appearances that are associated with the ways that the representation shows things as standing sensorily. Our hypothetical picture shows a chair, for example, precisely because anyone to whom things look a certain way that the picture shows things as looking thereby apparently sees a chair.

Extrapolating from the foregoing discussion yields the following tidy principle:[3]

(3.B)   A distinctively sensory representation shows an F which is G, on account of the ways that the representation shows things as standing sensorily, just in case there is some way that the representation shows things as standing sensorily which is such that anyone who has a sensation of that kind thereby seems sensorily to encounter an F which is G.

To put that principle into a slogan: *Scene-showing corresponds to seeming*. Recycling some terminology from the previous chapter, principle (3.B) tells us that the range of items that are scene-shown by a distinctively sensory representation is determined by the nature of the 'appearance-contents' belonging to the ways that the representation shows things as standing sensorily.

It is worth remarking that the claim that *scene-showing corresponds to seeming* posits a link between the items that are shown by a given distinctively sensory representation and the sensory appearances that inevitably accompany the types of sensations *that are singled out by the representation's content*. The principle does not itself posit a link between the items that are shown by a distinctively sensory representation and *the representation's own sensory character*. (Of course, that isn't to deny that those sorts of further connections may sometimes exist.) The principle thus does not entail that, say, the items that are shown by a picture are somehow related to what the picture itself looks like.

---

[3] Principle (3.B) merely illustrates a whole slew of related principles. So, for example, a distinctively sensory representation scene-shows an F standing in relation R to a G just in case, for some way that the representation shows things as standing sensorily, anyone who has a sensation of that kind thereby seems sensorily to encounter an F which stands in relation R to a G; a distinctively sensory representation scene-shows an F, a G, and an H standing in relation S just in case, for some way that the representation shows things as standing sensorily, anyone who has a sensation of that kind thereby seems sensorily to encounter an F, a G, and an H standing in relation S; and so on.

I have claimed that distinctively sensory representations single out types of sensations in a special way. But distinctively sensory representations are not just fancy lists of types of sensations. A picture may portray a visual episode from the inside, for example; or it may characterize the layout of the world around some viewpoint. In either case, though, the ways for things to look that are picked by the picture's content are used for further representational ends.

The next two sections identify two fundamentally different fashions in which distinctively sensory representations may show how things stand sensorily. The two modes of distinctively sensory showing correspond to two ways in which types of sensations may be used in ascribing properties. The resulting families of distinctively sensory contents are nonetheless alike, in that their members identify types of sensations in subjectively informative ways.

Sensation-characterizing

Chapter 1 distinguished subjective distinctively sensory representations (those which represent sensations) from objective ones (the rest). It also identified a particularly important family of subjective distinctively sensory representations: those which 'portray' sensations, by representing them from the inside. The current section presents an account of the special nature of the contents belonging to those distinctively sensory representations which portray sensations.

Use a tactile mental image to portray a tactile sensation. Your tactile mental image represents a tactile sensation from the inside because it shows things as feeling a certain way in the course of a tactile sensation. More fully, we have that *distinctively sensory showing comes from subjective informativeness*: the mental image's content singles out a certain way for things to feel, just in terms of what it is like to have a sensation in which things feel that way. But the image's content also characterizes a tactile sensation as being an instance of the type thereby singled out. The image therefore characterizes the represented sensation merely in terms of what the sensation is like for its subject. The tactile sensation represented by the tactile mental image is consequently represented 'from the inside'.

Generalizing, there are some distinctively sensory representations which 'show things as standing sensorily certain ways' in the following more specific manner: they show things as standing sensorily certain ways in the course of one or more sensations. Each distinctively sensory representation of that sort meets the following condition:

(3.C)   The representation's content singles out one or more sensation-types in a subjectively informative manner. And its content characterizes one or more sensations as being instances of those sensation-types.

Any distinctively sensory representation satisfying condition (3.C) is a *sensation-characterizing* distinctively sensory representation. Sensation-characterizing distinctively sensory representations portray sensations. (Note that the previous remark does not imply that sensation-characterizing distinctively sensory representations *only* portray sensations.) They are therefore subjective.

An important point: this book's Introduction briefly drew attention to the more or less complex sorts of contents which may belong to distinctively sensory representations. It also emphasized the relatively primitive variety of content which was to be our main concern: we were to focus on the representational facets of distinctively sensory representations deriving merely from the ways that they show things as standing sensorily.

A visual mental image, say, may serve to capture how things looked in the course of a particular past visual sensation that one enjoyed. But the identity of the relevant past visual sensation is not part of what one appreciates simply by virtue of one's grasp of how it is that the visual mental image shows things as looking 'in the course of a visual sensation'. Rather, one's mere appreciation of the way that the image shows things as looking in the course of a visual sensation corresponds to one's mere awareness, in the light of the visual mental image, of a certain sort of property that may be ascribed to visual sensations. (Similarly, you understand what my assertion that Nyirimana is a boy says 'about someone', simply because you associate my assertion with a property that may be ascribed to people.)

My talk of 'one or more sensations' in (3.C) therefore should not be taken as implying that sensation-characterizing distinctively sensory contents relate to specific sensations. Any bits of distinctively sensory contents that 'characterize sensations as being of certain types' should rather be understood to have the same kind of adjectival form as the meanings of predicates like '_ is a boy' or '_ is red'. For sensation-characterizing distinctively sensory contents proper merely capture properties that sensory episodes may possess.

For some later purposes, it will be helpful to employ some well-known metaphors when thinking about sensation-characterizing distinctively sensory contents. Frege introduced the idea that the adjectival meanings of predicates like '_ is a boy' contain 'gaps' that may be 'filled' using contents that denote specific objects; when the relevant gaps are filled, we end up with a content that ascribes a property to whatever is denoted by the content that has been used to fill the gap.[4] In the same vein, we may capture the adjectival nature of sensation-characterizing distinctively sensory contents by thinking of them too as having gaps, where the relevant gaps may be filled using contents that denote specific sensations.

So, for instance, use an auditory mental image to imagine apparently hearing a bell. Your auditory mental image shows things as sounding a certain way in the course of an auditory sensation: like *that*. Using a single underlining to symbolize a 'gap' that may be filled by contents that denote specific sensations, we might then regard the distinctively sensory content of your auditory mental image as being very roughly the following: things sound like *that* in the course of _.[5] The distinctively sensory content of the auditory mental image thus characterizes a property that auditory episodes may possess, without in itself ascribing that property to a specific auditory episode. The gappy nature of distinctively sensory contents opens up certain possibilities that will sometimes be exploited in later chapters; in particular, it will be relevant to Chapters 4 and 8.

---

[4] Frege [1891] 1997, [1892b] 1997, and [1904] 1980.

[5] The 'very roughly' needs emphasizing. The general form provided is an attempt to sketch, using linguistic resources, the nature of a certain distinctively sensory content; it should not be assumed that the relevant content really involves the conceptual materials mobilized by the language used in the text. (Similarly, one might attempt to give a rough idea of the form instantiated by the contents of the visual appearances which one is enjoying, by saying that 'here is how things look to me: there's an F with a G just next to it, and there's an H off to the right, and . . . ', without thereby committing oneself to holding that the concepts expressed by, for instance, 'next to' plus 'and' are really needed to capture the contents of the visual appearances being described; see the next chapter for further discussion of some related issues.)

Perspective-characterizing

Chapter 2 presented a general account of what it is for things to stand sensorily a certain way from a perspective:

(2.A)   A sensation-type T is a way that things stand sensorily from a perspective just in case T's appearance-content is true relative to the perspective.

More fully, suppose that T is a type of sensations. And suppose that the appearance-content of T is *things being thus*. That is, assume that, for any subject of a possible T-sensation, things seem sensorily to be *thus*; and assume that there is no more to the common way that things seem sensorily to be to the subjects of possible T-sensations than that, to each of them, things seem to be *thus*. Then T is a way that things stand sensorily from a perspective just in case things are *thus* relative to the perspective.

The previous section provided an account of what it is for a representation to show things as standing sensorily a certain way in the course of a sensation. The resulting account started from the obvious thought that what it is for things actually to stand sensorily a certain way *in the course of a sensation* is simply for the sensation to be an instance of the relevant type. But we may likewise use Chapter 2's claims about what it is for things actually to stand sensorily a certain way *from a perspective* to generate an account of what it is for a representation to show things as standing sensorily a certain way from a perspective.

Suppose, for instance, that you appreciate that a certain picture of a table shows things as looking some way. Then you might thereby take the picture simply to characterize what things are like around some perspective, by showing what things look like from there. Given the previous chapter's account of what it is for things to stand sensorily some way from a perspective, there is no mystery about what your interpretation of the picture would then involve.

For suppose that the visual appearances that form part of what it is for things to look the relevant way to a subject can be summarized by saying that they are visual appearances in which things look to be like *that*. Suppose, that is, that the appearance-content of the relevant way for things to look is *things being like that*. Then you might take the picture to characterize a perspective as being one relative to which things are like *that*. If you were to interpret the picture in that fashion, though, you would be taking the picture to show things as looking the relevant way from a perspective.

To extrapolate, there are some distinctively sensory representations which 'show things as standing sensorily certain ways' in the following more specific manner: they show things as standing sensorily certain ways from one or more perspectives. Each distinctively sensory representation of that sort meets the following condition:

(3.D)   The representation's content singles out one or more sensation-types in a subjectively informative manner. And its content characterizes the appearance-contents of those sensation-types as being true relative to one or more perspectives.

Any distinctively sensory representation satisfying condition (3.D) is a *perspective-characterizing* distinctively sensory representation.

In parallel with the previous section, perspective-characterizing distinctively sensory contents should be regarded as having gappy adjectival forms. (The identity of the particular historical occasion on which an audio recording was made is not part of what one grasps by means of one's mere appreciation of how it is that a playback of the recording shows things as sounding 'from somewhere', for instance. Rather, the latter corresponds to one's mere awareness, in the light of the playback, of a certain sort of property that may be ascribed to auditory perspectives.) The gaps in perspective-characterizing bits of distinctively sensory contents are to be filled by contents that denote specific perspectives, however, rather than by contents that denote specific sensations.

Note that, given the principle (3.D) just stated, a distinctively sensory representation may show things as standing sensorily a certain way from a perspective only if the relevant way for things to stand sensorily involves some accompanying sensory appearances. But maybe there are some modes of sensing which do not give rise to sensory appearances. Some people have suspected that bodily sensations like itches and stomach aches do not feature sensory appearances, for example. The form of showing how things stand sensorily identified by (3.D) thus may not be available for each and every variety of sensations; I will briefly return to this point towards the end of the chapter.

The current section and the previous one have identified two modes of showing things as standing sensorily certain ways. Each of the modes is associated with a distinctive kind of distinctively sensory contents. Yet those different sorts of distinctively sensory contents are alike in some obvious respects. For each of them uses subjectively informative modes of presentation to single out types of sensations. And the types of sensations thus picked out play predicative roles in each case; they are used to ascribe properties, either to sensations or to perspectives.

The core components of this book's theory of distinctively sensory content may therefore be summarized by combining a new slogan with one introduced earlier:

Distinctively sensory showing comes from subjective informativeness. And *distinctively sensory representations show things as standing sensorily certain ways, either from perspectives or in sensations.*

(It is perhaps worth explicitly noting, too, that the principle that *scene-showing corresponds to seeming* will be at least as important to this book as the two fundamental claims just sloganized.)

The second of those unsnappy catchphrases incorporates the unargued assumption that the two modes of showing things as standing sensorily certain ways distinguished above exhaust the options. One may produce, say, a visual mental image which portrays a visual sensation: that possibility is covered by the earlier account of sensation-characterizing distinctively sensory representations. And one may produce a visual mental image which just characterizes what things are like somewhere: a possibility that is covered by the earlier account of perspective-characterizing distinctively sensory representations. What else is there for visual mental images—and distinctively sensory representations in general—to do?

That question may reflect my own lack of imagination. It is therefore worth noting that this book's theory of distinctively sensory content may be regarded as being driven by two background thoughts. First, there is the thought that *distinctively sensory showing comes from subjective informativeness.* Second, there is the thought that distinctively sensory contents employ the types of sensations which they single out to ascribe properties to certain sorts of items. Maybe the property-ascriptions involved in distinctively sensory contents reach beyond the sensation-characterizing and perspective-characterizing ones discussed up to this point. But that would not obliterate the broad outlines of the approach to distinctively sensory contents being explored in this book.[6]

---

[6] It might be claimed that there are two ways in which a distinctively sensory representation may show things as standing sensorily a certain way in the course of a sensation: first, it

Explaining some constraints

Chapter 1 described a range of very general constraints applying to distinctively sensory representations. Each of the restrictions appears to reflect the distinctively sensory nature of distinctively sensory representations, as each of them corresponds to a limitation that applies to our sensory powers themselves. It is therefore reasonable to expect decent theories of distinctively sensory content to explain why distinctively sensory representations are subject to the relevant constraints.

The bulk of this section uses the theory of distinctively sensory content formulated above to explain why the restrictions noted in Chapter 1 apply to distinctively sensory representations. In fact, we will see that the theory explains why suitable limitations upon our sensory powers will always place corresponding constraints upon distinctively sensory representations. The various explanations that I am about to supply provide a significant initial illustration of the explanatory capacities of this book's ideas about distinctively sensory content.[7] The remainder of the chapter will provide further evidence of the explanatory powers of this book's theory of distinctively sensory content, by using the theory to vindicate the natural view that there can be both objective and subjective distinctively sensory representations.

1. Recall that distinctively sensory representations which show things are perspectival: they show the things that they show from perspectives, just as we seem to encounter scenes from perspectives in the course of sensory episodes. Produce a visual mental image which shows an empty chair, for instance. Your visual mental image shows the empty chair from somewhere. Why so?

---

may show things as standing sensorily a certain way in the course of a *mere sensation* (where the resulting characterization of a sensory episode is neutral on whether the episode is a genuine seeing, hearing, . . .); or, second, it may show things as standing sensorily a certain way in the course of a *perception* (where the sensory episode represented is thereby characterized as being a genuine seeing, hearing, . . . , so that the representation's portrayal of a sensory episode entails that the sensory episode occurs at a perspective from which things stand sensorily the relevant way). It makes no difference to anything that follows whether or not that proposal is correct.

[7] The explanations provided below greatly generalize and refine some similar explanations formulated specifically for pictures in Gregory 2010b.

Your visual mental image shows an empty chair because the way that it shows things as looking involves an empty chair, in accordance with the general fact that *scene-showing corresponds to seeming*:

(3.B) A distinctively sensory representation shows an *F* which is *G* just in case, for some way that the representation shows things as standing sensorily, anyone who has a sensation of that kind thereby seems sensorily to encounter an *F* which is *G*.

The way that your visual mental image shows things as looking is *Chair View*, let's say. One who has a *Chair View*-sensation thereby seems to see an empty chair.

Now, *distinctively sensory representations show things as standing sensorily certain ways, either from perspectives or in sensations*. Hence your visual mental image either has a sensation-characterizing content or it has a perspective-characterizing one.

Let's suppose, first, that your visual mental image has a sensation-characterizing content. Then (appealing to the account of sensation-characterizing contents provided earlier, in principle (3.C)) its content singles out *Chair View* in a subjectively informative manner and characterizes a sensation as being an instance of *Chair View*. The visual mental image therefore shows an empty chair by portraying a visual sensation in which an empty chair is apparently seen. But apparent seeings are perspectival. The visual mental image's showing of an empty chair is thus perspectival too.

Let's suppose, second, that your visual mental image has a perspective-characterizing content. Then (appealing to the account of perspective-characterizing contents provided earlier, in principle (3.D)) its content singles out *Chair View* in a subjectively informative manner and characterizes a perspective as being one relative to which *Chair View*'s appearance-content is true. The visual mental image therefore shows an empty chair by characterizing what things are like around a perspective, in a peculiarly visual fashion. The visual mental image's showing of an empty chair is thus again perspectival.

More generally, suppose that a distinctively sensory representation shows an *F*. The representation will show an *F* either by showing things as standing sensorily a certain way in the course of a sensation or by showing things as standing sensorily a certain way from a perspective.

But—as illustrated by the discussion of your visual mental image of an empty chair—in either case the representation's showing of an F will be perspectival.

2. Consider some distinctively sensory representation. We saw in Chapter 1 that the range of items which the representation shows will be limited in the following way: if the representation shows an F as being G, a subject could seem to encounter an F which is G by means of the sensory faculties involved in the ways that the representation shows things as standing sensorily. (Recall Alberti's comment that 'the painter is concerned solely with representing what can [apparently] be seen'.) Why so?

The previous representational limitation reflects the nature of our sensory capacities themselves. And this book's theory of distinctively sensory content makes it extremely easy to explain the noted restriction, just by appealing to corresponding points concerning sensations.

Suppose that some distinctively sensory representation shows an F which is G. We saw above that *scene-showing corresponds to seeming*. So, for some way that the representation shows things as standing sensorily, anyone who has a sensation of that kind thereby seems sensorily to encounter an F which is G. Hence an F that is G is the sort of thing which may apparently be sensed by means of some sensory modality to which the representation's distinctively sensory content is bound.[8] The limitation therefore follows.

---

[8] I have tacitly made a universal 'possibility assumption' here: for any sensation-type that is a way that a distinctively sensory representation shows things as standing sensorily, there could be some sensation in which things stand sensorily that way. (Produce a visual mental image. Doesn't it seem utterly evident to you that there could be a visual sensation in which things look the way that your visual mental image shows them as looking? More generally, it seems that any type of sensations whose instances may be identified in terms of their common subjective character has some possible instances. For suppose that some sensation-type may be picked out as encompassing exactly those sensations in which things are—as someone might put it—like *this*. Then how could there not be sensations in which things are like *this* for a subject? See Gregory 2010a for some further discussion of this sort of point about sensory mental imagery in relation to issues in modal epistemology.) If my universal possibility assumption is wrong, the explanation just provided only applies to those distinctively sensory representations that do satisfy suitable instances of the possibility assumption. But the resulting 'restriction' does not seem to be a problem. For suppose that a distinctively sensory representation shows an item by showing things as standing sensorily some way that things *cannot possibly* stand sensorily in the course of a sensation. Then why would one expect the representation's showing of the item to be constrained by the inevitable features of *possible* sensory encounters with things?

It is hardly more difficult to account for the final constraint that was identified in Chapter 1. Suppose that we are given a distinctively sensory representation whose content is bound to some sensory modality. And suppose that the representation shows an item as having some features which enable us to place it under a fairly general concept C. Finally, assume that the following holds: any sensory episode in which, by means of the relevant sensory modality, we apparently encounter an item having properties which enable us to characterize it as falling under C must amount to an apparent encounter with something of a comparatively more specific type. Then the representation's showing of an item which falls under C must likewise amount to the showing of something of a comparatively more specific type. Why?

To return to an example used in Chapter 1, consider a picture which shows a yellow ball placed between a red and a blue ball, where the balls are in a horizontal line. *Scene-showing corresponds to seeming*: hence for some way that the picture shows things as looking, anyone who has a sensation of that kind thereby seems to see a yellow ball, a red ball, and a blue ball lying in a horizontal line, with the yellow ball in the middle.

More particularly, though, the visual appearances that form part of what it is like to have a sensation in which things look the relevant way that the picture shows things as looking will be ones in which the red ball either looks to be on the left or looks to be on the right. (A red ball will not look to those who have visual sensations of the relevant kind merely to be *either* on the right *or* the left; visual appearances just are not like that.) As *scene-showing corresponds to seeming*, the picture must therefore either show the red ball as being on the left or show it as being on the right. Generalizing, the relative specificity of sensory appearances combines with the thesis that *scene-showing corresponds to seeming* to account immediately for the relative specificity manifested by distinctively sensory representations.[9]

3. The previous parts of this section showed how three highly general features of distinctively sensory representations may easily be explained using this chapter's theory of distinctively sensory content. Each of the features corresponds to a highly general characteristic of sensory episodes themselves. And, just intuitively, it seems clear that the corresponding

---

[9] The extrapolation in the text implicitly relies upon the universal possibility assumption stated in the previous footnote.

properties of sensory episodes are somehow responsible for the features of distinctively sensory representations.

The three explanations just provided respected that last point. In particular, the final two explanations—the ones provided under 2. above—shared a single overall form. First, a constraint C, applying to distinctively sensory representations in general, was noted. Second, it was recalled that *scene-showing corresponds to seeming*. Then, third, it was pointed out that possible sensory episodes themselves are subject to a constraint C^* that evidently corresponds to C. Finally, fourth, the fact that *scene-showing corresponds to seeming* was again employed, to argue that C^*'s application to sensations accounts for the fact that distinctively sensory representations are subject to C.[10]

That explanatory strategy may be applied to generate many further explanations. So, for example, distinctively tactile representations are unable to show negative facts; a tactile mental image, say, cannot show something as being not-*F*. (Tactile mental images can show things as having properties that are incompatible with other properties, but they do not thereby explicitly characterize the things which they show as *not having* the incompatible properties.) A similar point applies to distinctively visual and distinctively auditory representations. And if a distinctively visual representation shows two things from a single perspective, by showing things as looking a certain way, the representation must show the two items as standing in some spatial relationships.

Each of the representational handicaps just noted maps onto a corresponding sensory limitation. Something cannot look, sound, or feel by touch to be not-*F*; and if one seems to see two things at once then those things will look to stand in spatial relationships to one another. But *scene-showing corresponds to seeming*. The preceding restrictions in the ways that things may feel, look, or sound to be therefore immediately generate correlative representational limitations that apply to distinctively tactile, distinctively visual, and distinctively auditory representations. It is not hard to generate many further explanations that are cut from the same cloth.

In sum, the especially sensory nature of representations which show things as standing sensorily certain ways disables them in notable ways. For the sorts of scenes which the representations are capable of showing

---

[10] The universal possibility assumption stated two footnotes back will need to be invoked at this point.

depend upon the sorts of scenes which could apparently be encountered through the workings of suitable sensory powers. The theory of distinctively sensory content developed here allows us to expand upon and to substantiate those simple thoughts, by supplying a wide array of simple and elegant explanations of some of the most striking features of distinctively sensory representations.

Objective/subjective revisited

A distinctively sensory representation is subjective just in case it represents a sensation; otherwise, it is objective. As remarked in Chapter 1, it is very natural to think that there are both subjective and objective distinctively sensory representations. In fact, it seems that there can be subjective and objective distinctively sensory representations which show things as standing sensorily the very same ways. One may use a visual mental image of a table to portray a visual sensation in which a table is apparently seen, for instance. But it seems that one may also use a visual mental image that shows things as looking the same way merely to represent a table.

I suggested in Chapter 1 that the last point indicates the availability of two modes of showing how things stand sensorily. Can we use the theory of distinctively sensory content expounded above, with its delineation of two modes of showing things as standing sensorily certain ways, to explain how there may be both objective and subjective distinctively sensory representations? In particular, can the theory be used to explain how there may be an objective distinctively sensory representation which shows things as standing sensorily a certain way, where there may also be a subjective distinctively sensory representation which shows things as standing sensorily the very same way?

Use a visual mental image to imagine seeming to see a table. Let *Table View* be the way that your visual mental image shows things as looking. According to the theory articulated above, your visual mental image possesses a sensation-characterizing distinctively visual content: one that, first, identifies *Table View* in terms of what it is like to have a *Table View*-sensation and, second, characterizes a visual sensation as being an instance of *Table View*. Your visual mental image thus represents a *Table View*-sensation from the inside.

Next, use a visual mental image that shows things as looking the very same way merely to imagine a table. What has changed? The way that the visual mental image shows things as looking—*Table View*—has remained the same. The alteration lies in the representational labour that *Table View* is now being called upon to perform. For in this most recent case, *Table View* is simply serving to characterize how things are laid out around a perspective. To invoke the theory of distinctively sensory content presented above, your second visual mental image just, first, singles out *Table View* in a subjectively informative manner and, second, characterizes *Table View*'s appearance-content as being true relative to a perspective. The resulting visual mental image is therefore indeed an objective distinctively sensory representation, for the following reasons.

Consider *Table View*'s appearance-content: *things being thus*, let's say. I take it that whether or not things are *thus* relative to some perspective is not something which relates to how things are or are not within the mental life of a subject. But consider some perspective relative to which things are *thus*. There could be an empty counterpart of that perspective whose surrounding circumstances are just the same as those surrounding the initial perspective. Relative to that corresponding empty perspective, things would again be *thus*. For all of the non-mental aspects of the situations containing the initial perspective and its counterpart are just the same; and whether or not things are *thus* around a perspective has nothing to do with any mental matters.

Your latest visual mental image's characterization of a perspective as being one relative to which things are *thus* is therefore compatible with the perspective's being empty. So your visual mental image, in showing things as looking a certain way from a perspective, does not thereby represent a perspective at which a sensation occurs. Moreover, your visual mental image's characterization of things as being *thus* around a perspective does not require the presence of a sensation in any other place. For whether or not things are *thus* relative to a perspective has nothing to do with what things are like in the mental life of a subject. Your visual mental image therefore does not represent any sensations at all. Hence it is an objective distinctively sensory representation.[11]

---

[11] It is worth remarking parenthetically that your visual mental image's characterization of a perspective as being one relative to which things are *thus* is compatible both with the perspective's being occupied and with the presence of some sensations around the

For the record, the above argument generalizes to establish the following:

(3.E)   Suppose that distinctively sensory representation R shows things as standing sensorily certain ways from one or more perspectives, but does not show things as standing sensorily certain ways in the course of one or more sensations. And assume that each way T that R shows things as standing sensorily meets the following conditions: first, T's appearance-content is silent about mental matters; second, T's appearance-content could be true relative to some perspective p; and, third, there could be an empty but otherwise indiscernible counterpart of p. Then R is an objective distinctively sensory representation.

Plenty of distinctively sensory representations meet the conditions laid down in (3.E). So plenty of distinctively sensory representations are objective.

Principle (3.E) may be used to demonstrate that many pictures and visual mental images are objective distinctively sensory representations, for example. And it may be used to show that many playbacks of audio recordings and auditory mental images are objective distinctively sensory representations. Indeed, to pick up the theme of a discussion at the close of the previous chapter, it may be used to show that tactile mental images may be objective.

It should be emphasized that those last claims rest partly upon appeals to assumptions that do not themselves strictly form part of the theory of distinctively sensory content elaborated in this chapter. The reader is therefore free to accept the theory while rejecting the consequences that I have sought to use it to establish. But I think that the assumptions required for the derivation of those putative consequences are very plausible ones. The account of two modes of showing things as standing sensorily certain ways supplied above has therefore enabled me to meet another of the explanatory aims announced in Chapter 1: to account for the possibility of both objective and subjective distinctively sensory representations.

---

perspective. Hence, while your visual mental image of a table does not represent the *presence* of any sensations in the scene that it displays, it also does not represent the total *absence* of sensations from the displayed scene. Its content is, rather, neutral with regards to whether the scene incorporates any sensations. (See Gregory 2010d for some more on this point.)

To conclude this section, recall that sensation-characterizing distinctively sensory representations always represent sensations from the inside. It follows that objective distinctively sensory representations must merely show things as standing sensorily certain ways from perspectives. But suppose that there is some way for things to stand sensorily that does not involve any sensory appearances: it is not implausible to claim that itches do not feature sensory appearances, for example. As noted earlier in this chapter, no distinctively sensory representation can show things as standing sensorily that way from a perspective, because the relevant type of sensations is not associated with any sensory appearances, and hence does not have an appearance-content.

A range of distinctively sensory representations whose contents are bound to a certain sensory modality may therefore contain some objective cases only if the relevant sensory modality generates sensory appearances. Now, Martin argues that visualizings must always be imaginings of seeings, and his argument is examined in the following section. But he sets things up for his discussion by considering a sensory mental image of an itch, claiming fairly plausibly that 'in [sensorily] imagining the itch, one represents a situation of such a quality being instantiated, one represents the occurrence of such an experience'.[12]

I think that the plausibility of Martin's assertion—that imaginings employing sensory mental images of itches must thereby represent itchy episodes from the inside—largely derives from the plausibility of the thought that itches do not incorporate sensory appearances. For that last claim implies that itch images must always show how things feel in the course of sensations, rather than from perspectives. The claim accordingly also implies that itch images cannot be objective. Vision certainly does give rise to sensory appearances, however. So there is an important difference between sensory mental images of itches and mental visual imagery.

An argument blocked

The No Lookerless Looks argument formulated in Chapter 1 tried to demonstrate by main force the impossibility of objective distinctively sensory representations: it mistakenly assumed that anyone who holds that things stand sensorily a certain way from a perspective is thereby

---

[12] Martin 2002, 407.

committed to holding that a sensation occurs at the relevant perspective. But the No Lookerless Looks argument was a simplification of a more sophisticated line of thought concerning visualization, owed to Martin. To conclude this chapter, I shall briefly consider an interpretation of Martin's argument.[13]

Visual mental images show things in a perspectival fashion. But a visual mental image evidently need not show the very perspective from which it shows what it shows. And, even if the image does somehow show that perspective, the image's showing of the perspective does not itself make the perspective the one from which the image shows the scene that it displays. So why are perspectives inevitably implicated in visual mental images?

There is a parallel here with real visual episodes. In visual sensations, the special status of one's viewpoint—its status as the perspective from which one seems to see what one seems to see—does not derive from its apparently being seen by you. Rather, to quote Martin, 'the point of view from which one perceives is marked in one's visual experience through it being the point to which the objects perceived are presented—if one can fix the location of those objects, one [can] thereby determine the location of the point of view'.[14]

In the wake of that last comment, one might think that the role of the perspectives from which visual mental images show what they show is similarly derived from the fact that the images characterize the perspectives as being ones to which the shown scenes are presented.[15] But how is it that the image represents the shown scene as being 'presented' to a perspective?

Suppose that the visual mental image, in showing things as looking a certain way, portrays a sensation in which things look that way. Then the image surely does represent the scene that it shows 'as presented to a

---

[13]   Martin's argument is foreshadowed by some aspects of the discussion of visualization in Peacocke 1985. In that paper, Peacocke argues—in opposition to the claim in Williams 1973 that we can visualize unseen things—that for 'imaginings describable pre-theoretically as visualisations, hearings in one's head, or their analogues in other modalities . . . to imagine being φ in these cases is always at least to imagine from the inside an experience as of being φ' (Peacocke 1985, 22). Peacocke argues, too, that 'for such forms as "imagining a valley", we can say that to imagine an F is always to imagine from the inside an experience as of an F (or more weakly, an experience of a sort which might be enjoyed in perception of an F)' (Peacocke 1985, 23). Martin explicitly backs Peacocke as opposed to Williams (Martin 2002, 404). I am indebted to an anonymous referee for the *Philosophical Quarterly*, whose report on a draft of Gregory 2010d helped me to get a better grip on the mechanics of Martin's argument.
[14]   For both this quotation and the one in the previous sentence, see Martin 2002, 409–10.
[15]   Compare Martin 2002, 410.

perspective'. In particular, the image represents the shown scene as a sensing subject's apparent object of sight. We can thus smoothly explain the perspectival nature of visual mental images by assuming that visual mental images portray visual sensations. Martin says, more strongly, that the 'perspectival [nature] of visualising can only properly be explained by taking visualising to be the imagining of seeing'.[16]

The perspectival nature of some visual mental images is certainly to be explained in Martin's terms. In particular, consider a visual mental image that shows how things look in the course of a visual sensation. The scene shown by that image is characterized by the image as being 'presented to a perspective', in the strong sense that the scene is characterized by the image as being a sensing subject's apparent object of sight. But this chapter's theory of distinctively sensory content allows us to see that the perspectival nature of many other visual mental images is to be explained quite differently.

Consider a visual mental image that merely shows things as looking a certain way from a perspective. The image's distinctively visual content identifies a type of visual sensations in a subjectively informative manner; and it characterizes the type's appearance-content—*things being like that*, let's say—as being true relative to a perspective. The scene that is shown by the visual mental image—an ensemble of items that are like *that*—is thus represented by the image as 'presented to a perspective', in the very weak sense that the image's characterization of the scene is in terms of what things are like around a perspective.

Yet the visual mental image may nonetheless meet the various conditions that were identified in the previous section as guaranteeing the objectivity of distinctively sensory representations. More generally, there are many visualizings whose perspectival nature can properly be explained without taking the visualizings to be imaginings of sensations.[17] For their perspectival nature may simply be traced back to the fact that the visualizings feature visual mental images that show things as looking certain ways from perspectives.

---

[16] Martin 2002, 407. In a perhaps similar vein, Podro interprets Hegel as providing a 'treatment of painting as a projection seen from a given viewpoint and so implying the presence of the spectator' (1982, 24).

[17] Noordhof suggests, in his response to Martin 2002, that the perspectival nature of visualization derives from the fact 'that modes of sense perception . . . are phenomenally similar to equivalent modes of sensory imagining' (2002, 439), in that they merely involve related kinds of content. The reply to Martin's argument presented in the text provides one way of articulating that suggestion in more detail.

4

Applications and Extensions

Theories of content need to show that they are able to provide satisfying descriptions of relevant representational phenomena. This chapter explores various aspects of the theory of distinctively sensory content presented in Chapter 3, mainly to give the reader a better sense of the theory's flexibility and wide applicability. It is worth commenting that Chapters 5–8—which move away from pure theorizing about distinctively sensory content and into more well-explored areas—are independent of this one. Some readers may therefore wish to skip this chapter, hopefully to return to it at a later date.

The theoretical concerns of the preceding chapters were relatively rarefied and abstract. The current chapter will bring things down to earth a bit, by giving an initial illustration of how the ideas developed previously may be used to accommodate and illuminate some important representational phenomena as they are encapsulated in particular cases. Many of the examples used below are pictures, just because pictorial examples are the easiest cases to present in a book. But there is nothing in the treatments of the pictorial examples discussed shortly that does not generalize to cover suitably related non-visual and non-pictorial phenomena.

Here is the programme for what follows. The first few sections emphasize the important part played by *types* of sensations in this book's theory of distinctively sensory content, by considering various sorts of distinctively sensory representations that the theory is able easily to handle by invoking appropriate categories of sensations. That discussion leads into a brief survey of some of the forms of representational indeterminacy that the theory is also able comfortably to handle; following on from that, a slight refinement to the previous chapter's theory of distinctively sensory content is suggested. There are then some sections considering ways in which our understandings of distinctively sensory representations interact with our recognitional capacities and our conceptual repertoires.

The last two sections discuss some general issues about the nature of distinctively sensory contents. In particular, I discuss the relationships between this book's ideas about distinctively sensory content and issues relating to conceptual and non-conceptual contents. I also consider—all too inconclusively, alas, because of the magnitude of the philosophical issues involved—the relationships between distinctively sensory representations and verbal ones.

Familiar and unfamiliar types

I have claimed that *distinctively sensory showing comes from subjective informativeness*: distinctively sensory representations show things as standing sensorily certain ways by singling out types of sensations, merely in terms of what it is like to have sensations of those sorts. It follows that an individual is able to appreciate that a representation shows things as standing sensorily some way only if the individual is able to appreciate what it is like to have sensations of the relevant kind.

That implication seems right. We probably are not capable of appreciating what it is like to have, say, the sorts of echolocatory sensations enjoyed by bats and dolphins. Hence it seems unlikely that distinctively 'echolocatory' contents—as perhaps expressed by sensory mental images entertained by bats and dolphins—are ones that we are able to grasp. The range of distinctively sensory contents that we can grasp therefore does seem to be constrained by the range of sensory experiences whose subjective characters we are capable of appreciating. Yet there is, within the latter range, a very broad spread of more or less familiar ways for things to stand sensorily.

Consider Figure 4.1. Look for a moment at the face shown in Cooke's caricature. I hazard that you have never had a visual sensation in which things actually looked to you the way that you just grasped Figure 4.1 as showing things as looking. Yet you know what it would be like for things to look that way to a subject.

The idea that distinctively sensory representations 'show things as standing sensorily certain ways', when explained as in the previous chapter, thus does not mean that the contents of the distinctively sensory representations we may understand must doggedly reflect ways that things have in fact stood sensorily for us; nor does it mean that they must reflect the ways that things ordinarily stand sensorily for us. That is a good thing, as the ways that distinctively sensory representations show things as standing sensorily often

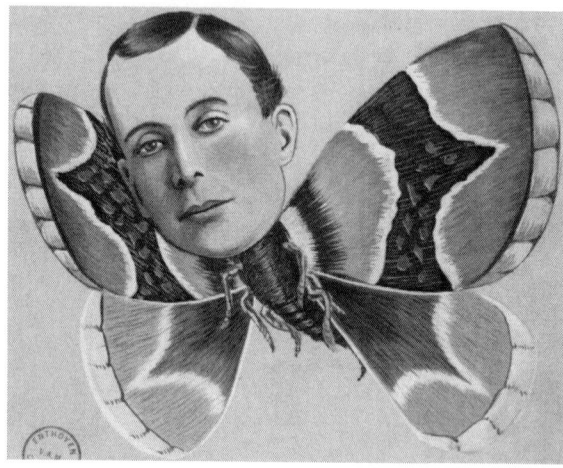

Figure 4.1. 'Poor Gaudy Butterfly': caricature of Arthur Lennard (1905), George Cooke[1]

are not ways that things typically stand or have ever stood sensorily for us. Indeed, distinctively sensory representations sometimes do educational work, by acquainting us with striking ways for things to stand sensorily.

The contents belonging to caricatures and expressionist paintings, for example, commonly involve ways for things to look that 'deform' more familiar ways for things to look. And one's views of such pictures may, in leading one to an awareness of what it would be like to have sensations in which things look those deformatory ways, enrich one's sense of the visual in numerous respects. You may realize, for example, that what it is like to enjoy visual sensations in which things look certain deformatory ways is in fact rather similar to what it is sometimes like for you in the course of visual episodes. One's appreciation of caricatures and expressionist pictures may thus make one aware of undercurrents sometimes running through one's own visual life; and many other examples of the same general sort could be cited.

Generality and specificity

Consider the sensation–type *Your View* whose instances are precisely those possible visual sensations that are subjectively indiscernible from the one

---

[1] © Victoria and Albert Museum, London.

which you are now having. The appearance-content of *Your View*—the shared way that things seem sensorily to be to the subjects of all possible *Your View*-sensations—amounts to no more nor less than the full way that things looked to you to be in the course of your own *Your View*-sensation. Imagine a distinctively visual representation which shows things as looking the very way that things just looked to you. Imagine, that is, that *Your View* is a way that things are shown as looking by some distinctively visual representation. The representation thereby shows a certain scene. And the level of detail incorporated in the shown scene will be precisely the level of detail incorporated in the visual appearances which formed part of your earlier *Your View*-sensation.

But the information which many of my supposed examples of distinctively sensory representations supply to us is considerably more denuded than that. Pictures, for instance, generally provide us with much more scanty information about the scenes which they show than visual appearances actually tend to provide us with about the scenes which we apparently see. The same sort of comments apply to auditory mental images, when their contents are compared with the contents of the auditory appearances that we actually enjoy. How can those points be squared with this book's theory of distinctively sensory content?

Like everything else, sensations come in more or less general varieties. We can identify the sensation-type *Your View De-Hued*, for example, whose instances consist of precisely those possible visual sensations which are either *Your View*-sensations or which differ from some *Your View*-sensation merely with regard to the hues of one or more things visible in the apparently viewed scene. *Your View De-Hued* is a more general sensation-type than *Your View*: its appearance-content is the same as *Your View*'s apart from being entirely non-committal with regard to the hues of the things in the posited scene.

Or, thinking back to your *Your View*-sensation, consider the sensation-type *One Outline From Your View*, whose instances are exactly those possible visual sensations in which something with *that* gross outline looks to be present *there*. *One Outline From Your View* is more general than both *Your View* and *Your View De-Hued*: its appearance-content consists of that fragment of *Your View De-Hued*'s appearance-content which posits the presence of something with a certain gross outline at a certain place.

But now suppose that there are distinctively visual representations that merely show *Your View De-Hued* and *One Outline From Your View* as being ways that things look from perspectives. Then the information which the representations provide about the scenes which they show is relatively bare, because of the generality of the appearance-contents belonging to those two sensation-types. The distinctively visual representation that just shows *Your View De-Hued* as being a way that things look from a perspective says nothing about the hues of anything in the shown scene; while the distinctively visual representation that just shows *One Outline From Your View* as being a way that things look from a perspective merely shows something having a certain overall outline at a certain position.

The earlier identification of ways that things stand sensorily with types of sensations therefore allows for distinctively sensory representations which show scenes in more or less schematic ways. For the ways for things to stand sensorily that may figure in distinctively sensory contents may be more or less general than one another. And this is an essential feature of the framework, without which it would not have a hope of applying as broadly as it is meant to. The next section relates those points to an example, and uses them to extract some further consequences.

Further discussion

Consider Figure 4.2. View some portion of Figure 4.2—one of the bits of the picture which shows the old man's right arm, say. In thus viewing the drawing, you have come to appreciate that the picture shows things as looking a certain way. Let's call that way for things to look *Right Arm View*. You could use a visual image to imagine a visual sensation that is an instance of *Right Arm View*.

Many of the possible visual sensations falling under *Right Arm View* will be subjectively discernible from one another, because of differences in the visual appearances which accompany the sensations. You could, for example, use a visual mental image to imagine a *Right Arm View*-sensation in which the reading man's robe looks to be dark brown. But, alternatively, you could use a visual mental image to imagine a *Right Arm View*-sensation in which the robe looks to be light brown.

Scene-showing corresponds to seeming: Figure 4.2 shows an *F* which is *G* just in case, for some way *T* that the drawing shows things as looking, any subject who enjoys a *T*-sensation thereby seems to see an *F* that is *G*. Hence the involvement of *Right Arm View* in Figure 4.2's distinctively

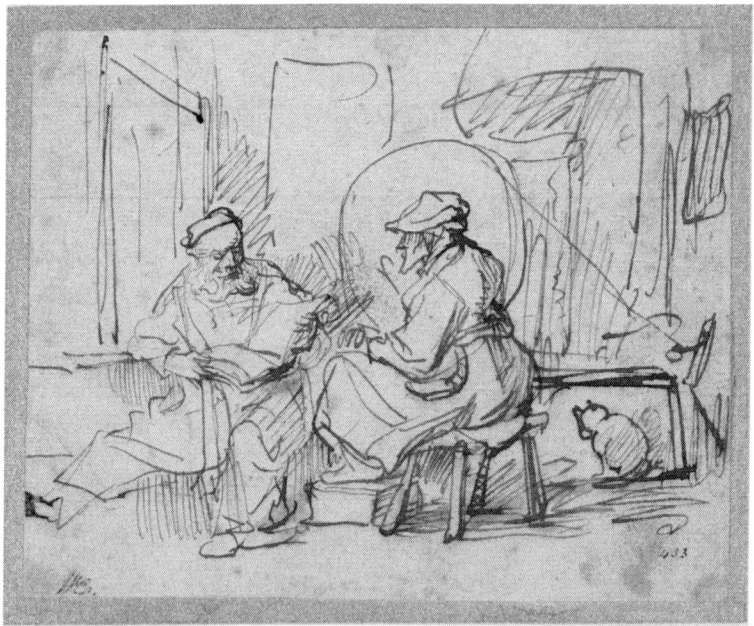

Figure 4.2. Old man (perhaps Tobit) reading to a seated woman (seventeenth century), copy after Rembrandt van Rijn[2]

visual content means that the picture shows a man having a certain property only if anyone who enjoys a *Right Arm View*-sensation thereby seems to see a man having the property.

But many of the possible sensations that are instances of *Right Arm View* are subjectively discernible in the sorts of ways noted previously. That point, combined with the thesis that *scene-showing corresponds to seeing*, implies that Figure 4.2's incorporation of *Right Arm View* within its content leaves open many of the features possessed by the reading man shown in the drawing. Figure 4.2 thereby shows neither a reading man whose robe is dark brown nor one whose robe is light brown, for example. And that is surely correct; just intuitively, Figure 4.2's overall sketchiness means that the drawing leaves undecided many features of what it shows, including the precise hue of the reading man's robe.

---

[2] © Victoria and Albert Museum, London.

The preceding comments relied upon what is, I think, the correct and most natural interpretation of Figure 4.2. But there are other less natural ways in which the drawing might be construed. Someone might insist, for instance, that the hue of a given patch of the reading man's robe should simply be identified with the hue of the portion of the drawing itself that shows the relevant patch. (This person would be like someone who insisted that black-and-white photographs should always be interpreted as showing black-and-white scenes, rather than as remaining neutral over the hues of the items contained in the shown scenes.)

That last rather perverse interpretation of the drawing raises various questions. Some of the questions are ones which my theory of distinctively sensory content cannot address without additional help. What explains the correctness of the interpretation which we actually employ, for example? And why does the alternative interpretation come much less naturally to us than the first one? (Are the differences merely conventional products of our own culture, or is there a deeper foundation for our interpretative tendencies?) Those queries—ones about how we interpret the drawing and about how it comes to possess its content—cannot be answered by a theory of distinctively sensory content alone.[3]

But the theory nonetheless allows us to isolate the crucial difference between the contents which the above two interpretations treat Figure 4.2 as expressing. The first and most natural interpretation—the one on which the drawing leaves out lots of colour-related information—identifies the types[4] of sensations figuring in Figure 4.2's distinctively visual content with ones whose appearance-contents say very little if anything about the hues of things. By contrast, the second interpretation identifies the relevant sensation-types with ones whose appearance-contents say rather a lot about hues. The theory thus at least allows us to respect the differences between the two interpretations, as well as to account for the manner in which one of them adds material to the other, even if it

---

[3] Many thanks to an anonymous referee for seeking clarification on these issues. Various treatments of picturing in the literature have invoked competing 'design-content correlations' (Lopes 1996, 153) of the sort discussed in the text: Goodman uses an interpretative scheme on which colours stand for their complements to argue against the claim that 'the most realistic picture is the one that provides the greatest amount of pertinent information' (1969, 35), for example, while Wollheim (1965, 24–5) appeals to the same interpretative scheme for different purposes. See Kulvicki 2010 for an interesting recent discussion of some of the questions raised by competing schemes of pictorial interpretation.

[4] The plural here is important; see the start of Chapter 7 for more discussion.

does not itself generate answers to all of the puzzles which the construals raise.

Drawings often provide compelling illustrations of the flexibility afforded to this book's theory of distinctively sensory content by its identification of ways for things to stand sensorily with types of sensations. But there are many other kinds of pictorial examples which could be used to make the same points: etchings, woodcuts, monochrome pictures, . . . could have been cited instead of the previous drawing. Indeed, many of the comments just made about Figure 4.2 apply even to quite 'lifelike' pictures, although (as we will see in Chapter 7) the lifelikeness of those pictures means that the ways that they show things as looking are relatively definite in some respects.

There is nothing especially pictorial or even visual about the phenomena just considered, of course. Use auditory mental imagery to imagine a bassoon playing the opening phrases of *The Rite of Spring*. Unless your inner ear is uncommonly acute, the ways that your auditory imagery shows things as sounding will not settle completely the nature of the bassoon's timbre, the precise volumes at which it plays the musical phrases . . . Those representational lacunae are akin to the indeterminacies that we have just seen to be present in the distinctively visual content of Figure 4.2. They correspond to differences in the possible hearings in which things sound the ways that your auditory mental image shows things as sounding.

Indeterminacies, from appearance-contents

As noted in the previous section, we may sometimes account for how distinctively sensory representations leave open features of the scenes which they show by invoking corresponding absences in the appearance-contents belonging to the ways that the representations show things as standing sensorily. Other forms of representational indeterminacy in distinctively sensory representations arise from indeterminacies in what appearance-contents do say about things.

Consider Figure 4.3. That picture shows various items, putting them some distance away from a perspective. But the distance standing between the things shown and the perspective is only very roughly defined; there are, for example, many values of n for which Figure 4.3 neither shows the

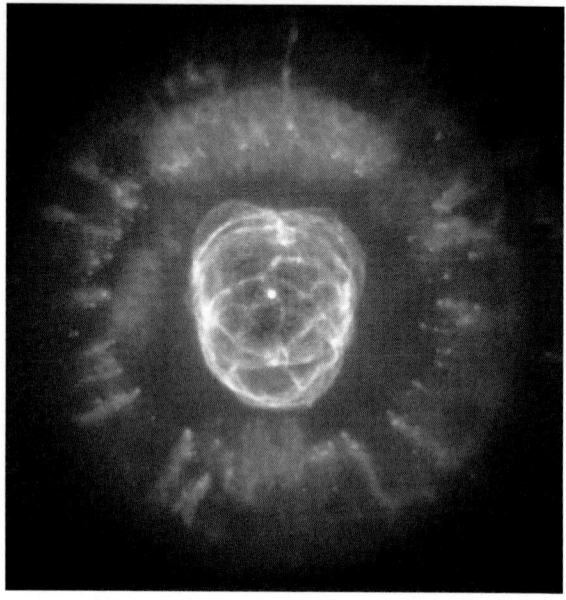

Figure 4.3. The 'Eskimo' Nebula (NGC 2392), NASA A. Fruchter and the ERO Team (STScl)

round central thing as being *n* centimetres away nor shows it as not being *n* centimetres away. As *scene-showing corresponds to seeming*, that fact about what the photo shows derives from the nature of the appearance-contents belonging to the ways for things to look which figure in Figure 4.3's distinctively sensory content.

Think of what it is like to gaze up into the heavens on a starry night. The stars look to be a long way away but the visual appearances which you enjoy do not purport to provide you with any very discriminating information about the distance which falls between the stars and your perspective. There are, in particular, many values of *n* for which the visual appearances neither verify nor falsify the claim that the stars are *n* centimetres away.[5] Equally, if things were to look to you some way that Figure 4.3 shows them as looking, you would not be provided with any

---

[5] See Siegel 2006, 378, for some similar remarks about a different case.

very discriminating distance-information by the visual appearances that you would thereby enjoy.

The appearance-contents belonging to the ways that Figure 4.3 shows things as looking thus involve distance-information that is rather rough. But the claim that *scene-showing corresponds to seeming* then implies that the roughness of the distance-information provided by the ways that Figure 4.3 shows things as looking is responsible for the corresponding lack of precision displayed by Figure 4.3's characterization of the whereabouts of what it shows.

There are many other ways in which the appearance-contents of ways for things to stand sensorily can be imprecise. Each of those modes of imprecision has the potential to result in correspondingly imprecise distinctively sensory representations. If I remove my glasses when looking into the middle to long distance, for instance, the ways that things look to me to be become indeterminate in various ways. If I form a visual mental image which shows things as looking one of those same ways from a perspective, the resulting visualization of a scene is afflicted with precisely the same blurry imprecision, which it inherits from the appearance-content of the way that the visual mental image shows things as looking. (Out-of-focus photographs often manifest the same sort of blurriness.)

To conclude this section, recall the sensation-type *Right Arm View* which we discussed in relation to the drawing reproduced as Figure 4.2. It is natural to think that the boundaries of *Right Arm View* are roughly defined. In particular, it is plausible that there are possible sensations which neither definitely are nor definitely are not instances of that type.

Suppose, though, that the vagueness of *Right Arm View*'s boundaries means that the nature of *Right Arm View*'s appearance-content is itself somewhat indeterminate with regard to some property *F*. More fully, suppose that it is neither definitely the case that anyone who has a *Right Arm View*-sensation thereby seems to see a man who is *F* nor definitely the case that someone who has a *Right Arm View*-sensation does not thereby seem to see a man who is *F*. Then, given that *scene-showing corresponds to seeming*, it will not definitely be the case that Figure 4.2 shows a man who is *F*, nor definitely the case that the drawing does not show a man who is *F*.

It is worth noting that the form of indeterminacy just mooted is quite distinct from the type of representational indeterminacy discussed in the previous section in relation to Figure 4.2. Those cases were exemplified by the way in which Figure 4.2 is definitely neutral with regard to certain

features of what it shows: the drawing does not settle the colour of the
reading man's robe, for example. But here we have something different, a
form of 'higher-order' indeterminacy. For we now have the apparent
possibility of instances in which it is indefinite whether or not a distinctively
sensory representation's showings are neutral with regard to various matters.

Relationships

Distinctively sensory representations frequently exhibit various forms of
multiperspectivalness and—to coin an ugly neologism for want of a better
word—multisensationality. A film may show things as looking many
different ways from a series of earlier and later perspectives, for example;
playbacks of audio recordings may perform an analogous auditory function. And it is easy for us to produce passages of sensory mental imagery
which show things as standing sensorily a range of distinct ways in the
course of earlier and later sensations. I can use olfactory mental imagery to
imagine an evolving sequence of smells, for example. Even still pictures
sometimes get up to the same sorts of tricks, as one can see by considering
Figure 4.4, a famous 'before and after' image.[6]

I take it that our appreciations of the kinds of temporal relationships just
cited are sometimes fundamental to our understandings of distinctively
sensory representations. So, one's knowledge that, say, a passage of film
shows how things looked from a particular sequence of past perspectives—
some perspectives lying near to Abraham Zapruder at about 12.30 p.m. on
22 November 1963, perhaps—is not something that is assured just by
one's ability to appreciate the ways that the film shows things as looking
'from some perspectives'. But it is very natural to think that one's appreciation of what the film displays, at that most basic level, will at least involve
an understanding of aspects of the temporal ordering holding among the

---

[6] All of the examples of multiperspectivalness and multisensationality just cited featured
non-simultaneous perspectives. But time is not of the essence here. Pictures can show the
different ways that things look at a single time from spatially separated perspectives, for
example: cubist pictures are often trotted out to make that point (see Clark 1999, 426,
footnote 31, for a brief survey of the genesis of the 'notion of Cubism involving the eye
"turning around" the object'). Indeed, pictures can show things as looking many ways at a
single time from the many perspectives that are located at a single place but which differ from
one another with regard to orientational factors; see the start of Chapter 7 for more on this
possibility, as it flows from the employment of some standard methods for the representation
of receding spaces.

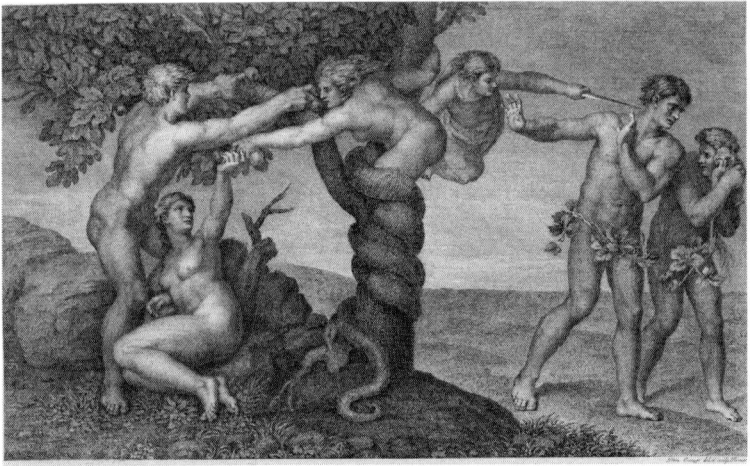

Figure 4.4. The Temptation and the Expulsion from Paradise, after Michelangelo's fresco in the Sistine Chapel (eighteenth century), Domenico Cunego[7]

perspectives to which the film's content relates: one will appreciate that *these* events—the passing cavalcade, the passenger's wave, . . . —came before *those* ones.[8]

Is there any way of incorporating those kinds of primitive spatiotemporal connections within distinctively sensory contents? Consider the perspective-characterizings involved in the ways that a certain distinctively sensory representation shows things as standing sensorily: suppose that the content characterizes a perspective as being one from which things look way *T* and that it also characterizes a perspective as being one from which things look way *U*. And let's suppose that part of what is involved in our grasp of the relevant content is an appreciation that the perspective from which the representation shows things as looking way *T* is, say, earlier than and to the left of the perspective from which the representation shows things as looking way *U*.

---

[7] © Victoria and Albert Museum, London.

[8] This might be denied; it might be claimed that one's mere grasp of the ways that, say, the Zapruder film shows things as looking from some perspectives does not itself provide one with any appreciation of spatiotemporal connections holding between the relevant perspectives. While that is a pretty radical position, it is a view which is also wholly compatible with the theory of distinctively sensory content defended here; to allow for it, one needs simply to ignore the additional complications relating to admissibility requirements which I am about to introduce.

Recall that, for the purposes of most of this book, I am focusing on the most primitive kind of content that belongs to distinctively sensory representations. It may be that some photograph shows how things once looked from some specific historic perspectives, for instance. But a person may understand the photo, by grasping that the photo shows things as looking certain ways 'from some perspectives', without appreciating the identities of the particular past perspectives whose surroundings are actually captured by the photo. My theory of distinctively sensory content handled that observation by treating distinctively sensory contents as expressing properties that may be ascribed to sensations or perspectives; and as thus being adjectival, in having gaps that are to be filled by contents that denote specific sensations and perspectives.

The distinctively sensory content that we are currently considering therefore does not relate to any specific perspectives; it too has a gappy adjectival form. How exactly, then, can our grasp of that content allow us to appreciate that 'the perspective' from which the representation shows things as looking way T is earlier and to the left of 'the perspective' from which the representation shows things as looking way U?

Our grasp of the representation's distinctively sensory content incorporates an appreciation that the representation captures certain properties that perspectives may possess. But the relevant properties of perspectives are not properties of spatiotemporally isolated perspectives. Rather, the content captures a potential arrangement of circumstances involving pairs of perspectives that are spatiotemporally related to one another in suitable ways. To provide a rough indication of the content's gappy adjectival form, the content characterizes things as looking way T from perspective _ and way U from perspective . . ., where perspective _ must be earlier than and to the left of perspective. . . .

We may add an extra ingredient to distinctively sensory contents to help us reflect those points. We can assume that distinctively sensory contents sometimes include *admissibility requirements*: constraints that define what counts as an acceptable way of filling the relevant content's gaps, where the constraints form part of what we appreciate upon grasping the relevant content. So, in the case just considered, the condition that 'perspective _ must be earlier than and to the left of perspective . . .' would be included within the relevant distinctively sensory content's admissibility requirements.

More generally, the inclusion of admissibility requirements within distinctively sensory contents enables the contents to impose spatiotemporal connections—and perhaps relationships of other sorts—upon the perspectives and sensations to which the properties expressed by the contents may properly be ascribed. Admissibility requirements thus provide a useful way of capturing various important phenomena involving distinctively sensory representations. They will not play any further role in this book's main text, however, although they will be deployed in some footnotes.

Up to now, this chapter has examined various features of the contents of distinctively sensory representations merely in the light of the ideas about distinctively sensory content presented in Chapter 3. But any account of the contents of distinctively sensory representations ought also to say something about how our understandings of distinctively sensory representations interact with other things; about their interactions with, for example, our recognitional capacities and our conceptual repertoires. The next couple of sections make some progress in that direction.

Descriptions of showings

Consider Figure 4.5, a drawing by Watteau. Here is the Victoria and Albert Museum's description of what the picture displays: '[s]eated figure of a man looking intently towards the right; he wears a cap trimmed with fur, and a dress which fits closely to the throat'.[9]

The thesis that *scene-showing corresponds to seeing* binds facts about what is shown by pictures having distinctively visual contents to facts about the contents of suitable visual appearances. In particular, the sorts of items that are shown by Watteau's drawing are those various types of things which would apparently be seen by any possible subject to whom things look some way that the picture shows things as looking. Now take the claim that the picture shows 'a cap trimmed with fur'. Given that *scene-showing corresponds to seeing*, we have the following: a cap trimmed with fur is shown by the picture only if, for some way that the picture shows things as looking, anyone to whom things look that way would thereby seem to see a cap trimmed with fur.

---

[9] From the web page <http://www.collections.vam.ac.uk/item/O246935/drawing/>, accessed at 13.38 on 8 May 2012.

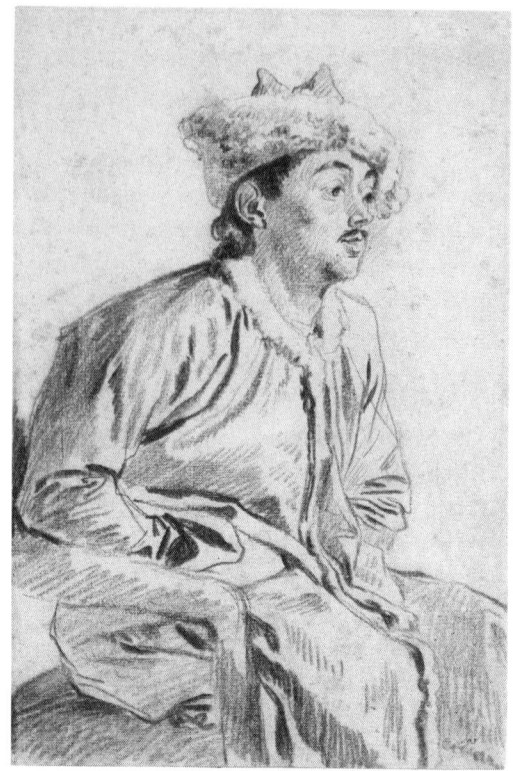

Figure 4.5. Seated figure of a man (late seventeenth–early eighteenth century), Jean-Antoine Watteau[10]

But—to return to an issue that has already briefly surfaced in earlier parts of this book—one might reasonably wonder whether someone could ever literally seem to see, say, 'a cap trimmed with fur'. Isn't the notion of a cap trimmed with fur more abstract than the concepts which most closely reflect the categories into which visual appearances put apparently present things? (Perhaps those categories cannot be captured using concepts at all; there is more discussion of this idea towards the end of this chapter.) Yet the earlier description of Figure 4.5 as showing a cap trimmed with fur is utterly anodyne. How is its mundaneness to be squared with the

---

[10] © Victoria and Albert Museum, London.

problematic nature of the claim that people may literally seem to see caps trimmed with fur?

The very outset of this book allowed for the possibility of distinctively sensory representations whose contents in the broadest sense are not exhausted by their distinctively sensory contents. Allegorical pictures have layers of content that do not simply derive from the ways that they show things as looking, for example. One might therefore be tempted to respond to the points just made by blandly insisting that we have here more of the same; by replying, that is, that the earlier claims about what Figure 4.5 represents just provide further illustrations of the way in which a picture may represent more than it shows.

On its own, though, that response is too curt. The assertion that this picture represents a cap trimmed with fur seems to be elementary in a way that, say, the statement that the picture shows 'a man who has paused for a moment to reflect upon his life' does not. How is the relative elementariness of the former to be recognized, other than by acknowledging that Figure 4.5 literally *shows* a cap trimmed with fur?

Review Figure 4.5. Form a visual mental image which shows things as looking, in the course of a visual sensation, some way that you have grasped Watteau's drawing as showing the man's head as looking. Suppose that, in the course of normal life, you were asked to describe what would seem to be seen by one who had a sensation of the kind—*Head View*, let's say—that you just imagined.

You would exhibit a peculiar form of preciousness if you were to insist that your response to that question must not mention the fur on the man's cap. And that is true even if visual appearances do not genuinely posit caps trimmed with fur. By contrast, consider the claim that a person to whom things looked your chosen way would seem to see 'a man who has paused for a moment to reflect upon his life'. There are many ordinary contexts in which someone who made that statement might be thought to be engaging in some rather tendentious mind reading.

It is therefore no wonder that, while we are happy enough with the claim that Figure 4.5 shows us a cap trimmed with fur, we are apt to regard the statement that the picture represents someone who has paused for a moment to reflect upon his life as more highfalutin.

For the principle that *scene-showing corresponds to seeming* tells us that, for any way which Figure 4.5 shows things as looking, Watteau's drawing shows those sorts of things which will apparently be seen in the course of any possible sensation in which things look that way. But *Head View* is a way that Figure 4.5 shows things as looking. And anyone who has a *Head View*-sensation will thereby 'seem to see a cap trimmed with fur'—or, at least, that is something that we are happy to say when we are not being terribly fussy about philosophical details. So Figure 4.5 does indeed 'show a cap trimmed with fur'—or, at least, that is something which we will usually allow ourselves to say.

By contrast, the claim that one who has a *Head View*-sensation will thereby 'seem to see a man who has paused for a moment to reflect upon his life' is less generally acceptable. The statement that Figure 4.5 'shows a man who has paused for a moment to reflect upon his life' will also be, correspondingly, less widely admissible. The different levels of evident acceptability belonging to the two earlier descriptions of what Figure 4.5 shows thus answer to the different levels of evident acceptability belonging to directly corresponding claims about the contents of visual appearances.[11]

More generally, there are contexts in which certain sorts of linguistic characterizations of the contents of sensory appearances are perfectly acceptable (although perhaps strictly speaking false). In those same contexts, though, correlative statements about the nature of what suitable distinctively sensory representations show should also be acceptable

---

[11] Wollheim (1998) presents a little thought experiment in which someone is taken to view a painting and is then asked about what she sees in the picture. The person accepts that she can see some columns shown by the painting as 'thrown down some hundreds of years ago by barbarians' (1998, 224). Wollheim takes the thought experiment to demonstrate the 'permeability to thought' (1998, 224) of seeing-in (the psychological capacity which Wollheim takes to be fundamental to the most basic form of pictorial representation). He claims that it is 'this feature that in turn accounts for the wide scope of seeing-in, wider, as we have seen, than that of seeing face-to-face' (1998, 224), presumably on the grounds that, say, some columns cannot literally look to have been thrown down some hundreds of years ago by barbarians. My own preferred response to this case would be to say that the envisaged picture does not literally show some columns as thrown down hundreds of years ago by barbarians, although it is fairly easy to explain why the claim that it does show some columns of that kind may be acceptable in certain contexts. More importantly, though, it is surely clear that we need to recognize a distinction between, first, the items that the picture represents simply on account of the ways that it shows things as looking and, second, the items that the picture represents in virtue of the ways that it shows things as looking and additional factors. No matter how one chooses to describe Wollheim's case, one therefore needs to recognize a division between the picture's distinctively visual content proper and the various parts of the picture's content that build upon, without themselves being part of, its distinctively visual content. (Many thanks to an anonymous referee for querying the relationship between the material in the text and Wollheim's discussion.)

(although, again, perhaps strictly speaking false). Given, however, that some of the expressions which we tend to use in describing the contents of sensory appearances are acceptable in an enormously wide array of contexts, it is therefore unsurprising that we do not wince at uses of those same expressions in specifying some of the most elementary representational properties of distinctively sensory representations. Indeed, I myself have repeatedly exploited that general point throughout this book, by describing distinctively sensory representations as showing things like tables, reading men and robes: those descriptions may strictly speaking have been false but they are also, in a sense, unproblematic.

Recognitional capacities

The previous section relied upon the banal point that, whether or not it is literally true to state that caps and fur figure in the contents of visual appearances, it is at least typically acceptable by ordinary standards to assert that we sometimes seem to see caps trimmed with fur. Yet suppose that visual appearances never do literally posit, say, caps. Then why do we rarely look askance upon people who claim to seem to see caps? What relationship between the contents of some visual appearances and the concept of being a cap makes it fair to say, in a given case, that the appearances are ones in which a cap seems to be in view?

There are probably many different relationships which can properly be cited in reply to questions like that last one. But it will be worth logging one pertinent sort of case here, because of its relevance to some further issues of interest.

Suppose that, one day, I peep into a joiner's workshop and seem to see something that I recognize by sight as being a bandsaw. Then, under ordinary circumstances, I would happily say that I seemed to see a bandsaw in my glimpse of the workshop. But suppose that, on the same occasion, I seem to see something which would be classified as a biscuit jointer by those in the know, although I am not able to recognize it as such. Then—assuming my continued ignorance of what biscuit jointers look like—I would not ordinarily accept the claim that I seemed to see a biscuit jointer (even though I might not positively reject that claim). Our capacities to classify things conceptually by means of their visual appearances thus often play an important role in determining our responses to claims about what we 'seem to see'.

More generally, suppose that one knows what *F*s look like. But suppose that one does not know what *G*s look like. And suppose that one is aware of what it is like to have a sensation in which things look a certain way *T*. Then one's awareness of what it is like for things to look that way to someone will typically combine with one's knowledge of what *F*s look like, to enable one to assess whether or not one of the things which seems to seen by one who has a *T*-sensation may acceptably be classified as an *F*. One's ignorance of what *G*s look like, however, will generally prevent one from assessing whether or not any of the things which seem to seen by one who has a *T*-sensation may acceptably be classified as a *G*. Analogous points apply to all of those other types of sensations which feature sensory appearances.

Philosophers discussing pictures have often noted that our knowledge of the visual appearances of things commonly enables us to classify conceptually the things which pictures show. Hopkins, for example, states that '[g]eneral competence with depiction and knowledge of the appearance of [*F*s] suffice for the ability to interpret depiction of [*F*s]', and '[g]eneral competence with depiction and knowledge of the appearance of [*F*s] are necessary for the ability to interpret depiction of [*F*s]'.[12]

Similar remarks apply to other sorts of distinctively sensory representations. Suppose that one knows what working bandsaws sound like and that one appreciates how some playback of an audio recording shows things as sounding. Then one will normally be able to tell whether or not the playback presents a bandsaw at work. But someone who does not know what working bandsaws sound like will not be able to tell, just by hearing the playback, whether or not a working bandsaw is one of the things that the playback presents. Is the theory of distinctively sensory content

---

[12] Hopkins 1998, 31; see Chapter 6 for more discussion of 'depiction'. (Hopkins's exact formulations are 'General competence with depiction and knowledge of the appearance of O (be it a particular *a* or merely *a*, but no particular, F-thing) suffice for the ability to interpret depiction of O' and 'General competence with depiction and knowledge of the appearance of O are necessary for the ability to interpret depiction of O'.) Schier 1986 provides the most extended treatment of the phenomena cited in the text (see, for instance, pp. 43–9 of Schier's book); Schier in fact seeks to build a theory of the nature of depiction itself upon the phenomena (see Chapter 6 for some discussion of Schier's ideas). See also, for example, Peacocke 1987, 395; Wollheim 1987, 77; Budd 1993, 170; Lopes 1996, 70–1.

articulated in the previous chapter able to help us account for those sorts of points?

Our appreciation of the ways that Figure 4.5 shows things as looking leads us to allow that one of the things shown by Figure 4.5 may acceptably be described as a cap trimmed with fur. How so? Reconsider the sensation-type *Head View* discussed above. *Distinctively sensory showing comes from subjective informativeness.* Our appreciation that *Head View* is a way that Watteau's drawing shows things as looking thus calls upon our ability to identify *Head View* in terms of what it is like to have a sensation in which things look that way.

Now, we know what caps trimmed with fur look like. And we are aware of what it is like to have a *Head View*-sensation. Hence we have the wherewithal to judge correctly that anyone who has a *Head View*-sensation will seem to see something that may acceptably be classified as a cap trimmed with fur. But *scene-showing corresponds to seeming.* In particular, Figure 4.5 shows anything which would seem to be seen by anyone who has a *Head View*-sensation. Our understanding of what it is for pictures to show things means that we are therefore also able to judge that one of the things that is shown by Watteau's drawing may acceptably be categorized as a cap trimmed with fur.

That line of argument generalizes straightforwardly, to explain why an awareness of what *F*s look or sound or feel or . . . like usually provides one with the ability to tell whether suitable types of distinctively sensory representation show *F*s. A similar line of argument may be employed to explain why an ignorance of what *F*s look or sound or feel or . . . like tends to prevent one from being able to tell whether appropriate varieties of distinctively sensory representations show *F*s. And the generality of the resulting explanations, which derives from their use of a general theory of distinctively sensory content, is important. For there is nothing essentially pictorial, or even visual, about classificatory interactions between our recognitional capacities and distinctively sensory representations.

This section explored some of the ways in which distinctively sensory contents may engage with our conceptual capabilities. But are distinctively sensory contents ever themselves conceptual? And how do they relate to the contents expressed by, say, sentences of natural languages? I will not attempt to offer definitive responses to those questions: I do not need to answer them for the purposes of this book; and, as we will see, their resolution must anyway derive from replies to various broader questions that I cannot reasonably hope properly to address here. The main aim of the last couple of sections in this chapter is therefore simply to delineate some of the complex factors that will need to be taken into account in resolving questions like the ones just posed.

Further correspondences

One notable recent debate in the philosophy of perception has concerned whether the contents of sensory appearances are non-conceptual.[13] That debate's focus, on seeking better to understand the nature of a variety of peculiarly sensory information, fits very nicely with my own focus in the current book. What are the relationships between this book's theory of distinctively sensory content and arguments over the conceptual or non-conceptual natures of the contents of sensory appearances? As we will see shortly, the theory itself is neutral on the outcomes of the latter debates. But the thesis that *scene-showing corresponds to seeming* nonetheless implies that the debates' outcomes will settle fundamental questions about the natures of distinctively sensory contents.

There are various ways of interpreting the statement that the contents of sensory appearances are 'non-conceptual'. On one reading, for instance, it amounts to the claim that a sensing subject may enjoy some sensory appearances which possess a given content even though the subject does not possess the concepts which would be required for her to have, say, a belief with that same content.[14] But, on another construal, it amounts to the statement that the contents of sensory appearances are fundamentally different from conceptually composed contents.[15] Just as it is natural to wonder whether the contents of sensory states are non-conceptual in various ways, it is natural to ask whether the contents of corresponding forms of distinctively sensory representation are non-conceptual in those same ways.

---

[13] Gunther 2003 is a helpful anthology of relevant papers.

[14] Martin 1992, for example, argues that sensory states have non-conceptual content in this sense.

[15] See Heck 2007 for a recent discussion that argues that sensory states have non-conceptual content in this sense. The obvious thought here is just that '[p]erceptual experience has a richness, texture and fineness of grain that beliefs do not and cannot have' (Bermúdez 1995, 335).

So, Martin argues that a subject may enjoy some visual appearances with a certain content even though the person does not have the concepts which would be needed for her to have a belief with that content. In particular, Martin points to the apparent possibility of someone's realizing that she once seemed to see a twelve-sided die in the course of a board game even though she did not possess the concept of twelve-sidedness at that earlier time.[16] Similarly, though, it seems that the person might realize that she once saw and understood a photograph which showed a twelve-sided die, although she did not have the concept of twelve-sidedness when she viewed the photo.

Let's suppose, for the sake of argument, that Martin is wrong; suppose, that is, that the contents of the sensory appearances that one can enjoy are constrained by the concepts that one possesses. Now consider some subject who lacks the concept of twelve-sidedness. That subject presumably will be unable to appreciate what it is like to seem to see a twelve-sided die, on account of the assumed limitation in her conceptual repertoire. But if the subject is unable to appreciate what it is like to seem to see a twelve-sided die, she will be unable to grasp the distinctively visual content of, say, a picture which shows a twelve-sided die. For the previous chapter's theory of distinctively sensory content tells us that, for any picture that shows a twelve-sided die, one may appreciate the ways that the picture shows things as looking only if one is able to appreciate what it is like to have sensations in which things look those ways. If the range of visual appearances that we can enjoy are constrained by the concepts which we possess, then, so too is the range of distinctively visual contents that we can grasp.[17]

---

[16] Martin 1992, 753–5.

[17] More fully, consider a picture that shows an F. *Scene-showing corresponds to seeming*; so, for some way W that the picture shows things as looking, part of what it is for things to look that way to a person is for the person apparently to see an F. But one may therefore appreciate what it is like to have a W-sensation only if one is able to appreciate what it is like to seem to see an F. *Distinctively sensory showing comes from subjective informativeness*: our picture's content identifies W in terms of what it is like to have a sensation in which things look that way. Hence one may grasp the picture's distinctively visual content only if one can appreciate what it is like to seem to see an F. But the thesis that one may seem to see an F only if one has the concept F presumably generalizes to imply that one may appreciate *what it is like to seem to see an F* only if one has the concept F. So the thesis that one may seem to see an F only if one has the concept F also implies that one may grasp the distinctively visual content of our initial picture only if one has the concept F.

More generally, there are lots of tough philosophical questions about whether the sensory appearances that we enjoy are subject to various broad constraints. Are the contents of visual or auditory sensations non-conceptual in Martin's sense? Do the contents of visual and tactile appearances overlap? Do the contents of sensory appearances ever make reference to specific individuals, so that the veridicality of some sensory appearances might require the presence of a certain individual as opposed to its qualitatively indiscernible twin? Philosophy being what it is, those questions are not ones about whether the contents of the relevant sensory appearances just happen to be subject to particular limitations. They are, instead, ones pertaining to whether the contents of the sensory appearances essentially suffer from the relevant restrictions.

Yet suppose that the contents of the sensory appearances associated with a specific sensory modality M are intrinsically limited in some respect. How could we appreciate what it is like to enjoy sensory appearances owed to M which are not limited in the relevant manner? The argument rehearsed a few moments ago (in relation to pictures showing twelve-sided dice) may then be adapted to demonstrate the following: any distinctively sensory representation that we can comprehend and that does some distinctively sensory showing which is bound to M will be subject to the same limitation as the sensory appearances produced by M.

The theory of distinctively sensory content presented in Chapter 3 thus implies that the answers to fundamental philosophical questions about the constraints applying to the contents of sensory appearances will have immediate consequences for correspondingly fundamental questions about the constraints applying to distinctively sensory contents.

So, suppose that the contents of visual and auditory appearances are inevitably non-conceptual, in that they always differ fundamentally from conceptually composed contents. The contents of distinctively visual and distinctively auditory representations will therefore be non-conceptual in the same sense. But suppose, instead, that the contents of visual and auditory appearances are conceptual, in that the range of concepts possessed by a subject restrict the range of visual and auditory appearances whose subjective character the subject is capable of appreciating. Then the contents of the distinctively visual and auditory representations that the subject may understand will be conceptual in just the same way.

All that is exactly as it should be. One would expect facts about the ways that distinctively sensory representations may show things as standing sensorily ultimately to depend upon facts about the ways that things may stand sensorily. There are consequently many deep questions about distinctively sensory contents whose solutions are beyond the scope of this book, just because their answers are tied to more basic issues in the philosophy of perception which I cannot hope now to resolve.

For that reason, this book's theory of distinctively sensory content cannot pretend to be a complete account of the nature of distinctively sensory contents. Like most theories, the one being developed here leaves certain details to be filled in at a later date. In particular, the theory treats general facts about the nature of what may be shown by distinctively sensory representations as parasitic upon general facts about the nature of sensory appearances; at which point it passes on the baton to theories of sensory experience. But while the theory therefore is not omnipotent, it is far from impotent: this chapter and the previous one have provided some evidence of its explanatory capabilities, and plenty more is provided below.

Language

We tend naturally to regard linguistic representations as being very different from, say, pictures. Our suspicion that there are significant differences between sentences and pictures partly derives from our sense that there are fundamental dissimilarities in the ways that we come to grasp the contents of pictures and sentences. The very process of looking comprehendingly at a picture just feels unlike the process of listening comprehendingly to someone's speech, or of reading a passage of text.

Some of the crucial differences between linguistic representations and restricted varieties of distinctively sensory representations thus arise from the ways in which we grasp the representations' contents. And this book's theory of distinctively sensory content cannot illuminate those contrasts without further help; to account for them, the theory would need to be supplemented by ideas concerning, say, how distinctively sensory representations express their contents.

Our awareness of important differences does not just seem to relate to the means by which pictures and sentences express their contents, though. For there is a sense in which a picture of, say, a house and a visual mental image of one are more like one another than they are like a typical written description of a house. Yet our eyes clearly play a larger role in our comprehension of the written text and the picture than they play in our grasp of the content of the visual mental image. Might this second dimension of difference be owed to the fact that verbal descriptions of houses, and verbal representations more generally, cannot possess distinctively sensory contents?

The question whether verbal representations can possess distinctively sensory contents is extremely general. To answer it properly, one would need somehow to take into account the full spectrum of merely possible sensory modalities along with the complete range of merely possible languages. One might restrict one's attention to the sorts of sensory powers that we possess along with the sorts of languages that we speak, of course. Yet to do that would hardly help: to my knowledge at least, a compelling account of the nature of the contents that may be expressed using typical human languages is not to hand.

All is not lost, however. The earlier parts of this book posited various connections between distinctively sensory representations and ways for things to stand sensorily. The discussions thus implied that linguistic distinctively sensory representations are possible only if linguistic representations are capable of standing in those same relationships to types of sensations. While I am unable to prove that verbal representations and sensation-types certainly cannot stand in the relevant relationships, I suspect that—perhaps with the exception of some special cases featuring demonstratives, discussed shortly—many people would be attracted to the view that they cannot. And, for people who are attracted to that view, the thesis that standard verbal representations cannot possess distinctively sensory contents should be correspondingly appealing.

To make things more tractable, let's ignore the profusion of actual and merely possible sensory modalities that we do not possess. The theory presented in the previous chapter claimed, first, that *distinctively sensory showing comes from subjective informativeness*; and it claimed, second, that *distinctively sensory representations show things as standing sensorily certain ways, either from perspectives or in sensations*. Recall, too, that a way for things to stand sensorily is identified in a subjectively informative manner just in case the type is identified merely in terms of what it is like to have a sensation in which things stand sensorily that way.

Some representations may therefore express distinctively sensory contents only if they meet the following two conditions. First, the representations can single out *subjectively unified* ways for things to stand sensorily: sensation-types that encompass all and only those possible sensations that share some 'what-it's-like-ness'. And, second, the representations can identify subjectively unified ways for things to stand sensorily merely in terms of what it is like to have sensations of those sorts. How do verbal representations fare in relation to those conditions? Let's start by considering some cases featuring demonstratives.

Things look like *this* to me right now. Consider the sensation-type encompassing just those possible sensations in which things look like *this* to someone. That sensation-type is subjectively unified. Yet one might also think that the description 'the sensation-type encompassing just those possible sensations in which things look like *this* to a subject' identifies a type of sensations in terms of what it is like to have a sensation of that sort: it is to have a sensation in which things look like *this*!

It is easy to produce similar examples involving demonstrative references to the ways that distinctively sensory representations show things as standing sensorily. Produce a tactile mental image, for instance. You may use the image to pick out the sensation-type encompassing just those possible sensations in which things feel like *that* to someone.

Such demonstrative-based verbal descriptions of ways for things to stand sensorily may seem to clear the path to linguistic distinctively sensory representations, by identifying subjectively unified types of sensations in subjectively informative ways.[18] Now, there may be good strategies for blocking those putative cases; on the other hand, though, perhaps there aren't. No matter. After all, uses of demonstratives promise to allow one verbally to express *any* variety of contents possessed by some type of representations whose instances one is able sometimes to indicate. The idea that we might verbally express distinctively sensory contents using demonstratives whose contents are parasitic upon the contents of indicated distinctively sensory representations hardly seems troubling.

The question whether we may express distinctively sensory contents using words looks more interesting once demonstratives are removed from the scene, though. The previous chapter featured the start of a verbal

---

[18] The role for demonstratives being considered in the text is reminiscent of a role that they have played in some debates over non-conceptual contents, where they have been used as a mechanism for bringing putatively non-conceptual phenomena within the realm of the conceptual: see, for instance, McDowell 1994, 82–4 (see also Heck 2000 for discussion).

description of the way that things once looked to me: 'I seem to see a computer screen with a loudspeaker next to it, both of which stand in front of a wall that has lots of pictures by children stuck to it; the computer screen has some letters of the alphabet on it . . . '. Could the resulting description have identified, first, a subjectively unified way for things to stand sensorily simply, second, in terms of what it is like to have sensations of the relevant kind?

Take the first of those two conditions. There is no subjective character which is common to precisely those possible visual sensations in which 'one seems to see a computer screen with a loudspeaker next to it, both of which stand in front of a wall that has lots of pictures by children stuck to it, and where the computer screen has some letters on it'. Just consider, for instance, the variations in the apparent distances between screen and speaker, in the shapes of the speaker . . . which are encompassed by the family of possible visual sensations in which things look the way described.

One could greatly add to the previous description. And one could seek to enhance it in other ways: one could rid the description of talk of 'computer screens', for example, and resolve only to use especially simple descriptive terms for speaking of particularly simple visible features of the environment. But—or so I am tempted to think, anyway—the resulting descriptions would still fail to identify subjectively unified ways for things to look. For the levels of subjective variation in the possible sensations covered by the descriptions would continue to mean that those sensations do not form subjectively unified kinds. If one is tempted by that thought, however, one should deny that the revised descriptions would be distinctively sensory ones.

Consider next the second of the two constraints upon distinctively sensory representations stated above: that distinctively sensory representations must be able to identify subjectively unified sensation-types in terms of what it is like to have sensations of those kinds.

Suppose that one uses demonstrative-free language to single out a type of visual sensations in which 'one seems to see a computer screen with a loudspeaker next to it, both of which stand in front of a wall that has lots of pictures by children stuck to it; the computer screen has some letters on it . . . '. And suppose—maybe *per impossibile*—that the possible instances of the specified type are just those possible sensations that share a certain subjective character. Could it be that anyone who understands that description thereby identifies a sensation-type simply in terms of what it is like to undergo sensations of the relevant kind?

To address that question properly, I would need to enter into detailed discussions of many other questions that are well beyond this book's remit. I would need to examine the relationships between our sensory powers and what is required of us if we are to grasp certain kinds of verbally expressible contents, for instance. But, for what it is worth, I cannot myself envisage a demonstrative-free verbal description of a way that things look to a subject that would fit the bill; that is, one that would isolate a subjectively unified family of visual sensations by just homing in upon the very subjective character which the sensations all share. Anyone who shares that hunch—and it is merely a hunch—should again be inclined to deny that linguistic representations can be distinctively sensory ones.

It should also be noted that one might allow for linguistic distinctively sensory representations while fully acknowledging the specialness of suitable categories of non-verbal distinctively sensory representations. We can accept that there are verbal descriptions whose distinctively visual contents overlap with the distinctively visual contents of pictures, for instance, without being forced to the absurdity that the verbal descriptions are themselves pictures. For there is clearly more to literal picturing than the mere possession of distinctively visual contents: visual mental images also have distinctively visual contents, for example. More specifically, it seems obvious that pictures possessing distinctively visual contents express their distinctively visual contents in especially pictorial ways.

To conclude: there are many important general issues about the relationships between the contents of linguistic representations and distinctively sensory contents that this book has no hope of finally resolving. But the theory of distinctively sensory content developed here enables us to make some partial progress on those matters, by isolating significant conditions which linguistic distinctively sensory representations would have to meet. The theory may thus enable one to arrive at a firmer sense of the ways in which one's beliefs about language, sensations, and appropriate sorts of non-verbal representations should interact, even if the theory alone cannot tell us everything about how those phenomena actually relate to one another.

5

Mental Images

Chapter 3's theory of distinctively sensory content stated that *distinctively sensory showing comes from subjective informativeness*. It also stated that *distinctively sensory representations show things as standing sensorily certain ways, either from perspectives or in sensations*.

Part of the support for the theory stems from its status as an appealing theoretical refinement of the simple thought that there is a significant unity to the contents belonging to those representations that show things as standing sensorily certain ways. Another part of the theory's support comes from its explanatory and descriptive virtues. In particular, the previous two chapters showed how the theory may be used to account for numerous features of distinctively sensory representations.

The theorizing about content which filled the first part of this book was very general, however; although the previous chapter contained some pictures, its investigations paid scant attention to the differences that hold pictures apart from many other families of distinctively sensory representations. The body of earlier work on distinctively sensory representations takes a less broad approach than the one developed above. Its authors tend to concentrate on questions about how particular kinds of distinctively sensory representations express their distinctively sensory contents, rather than upon theorizing about distinctively sensory content per se.

The following three chapters make direct contact with more common concerns. They examine some restricted groups of distinctively sensory representations in the light of the theory of distinctively sensory content developed previously; and they show how the framework may be used to generate the sorts of conclusions that have been the targets of earlier work on distinctively sensory representations. The next few chapters thus provide further support for this book's theory of distinctively sensory content, by illustrating how it may be employed to shed light on relatively restricted ranges of distinctively sensory representations.

In particular, the following thought will be important to some arguments in both this chapter and the next one: that we may use the thesis that *distinctively sensory showing comes from subjective informativeness* to generate conclusions about how certain sorts of representational media may be exploited to express distinctively sensory contents.

The imagery debate

The last few decades have seen an explosion of empirical studies of sensory mental images, and of visualization in particular. Those studies have thrown into relief a host of important questions about the phenomena: questions about the nature of the representational formats utilized in episodes featuring sensory mental imagery, for example, and about the nature of the neurological resources which the episodes exploit. The precise bearing of various bodies of empirical evidence upon such topics is the focus of an important interdisciplinary controversy—more properly, family of controversies—involving philosophers, psychologists, and neurophysiologists, one that is often known simply as 'the imagery debate'.[1]

Kosslyn and Pylyshyn are the most well-known participants in the imagery debate; the disagreements between those two thinkers have to a large extent set the very terms of the ensuing arguments. As we will see at more length below, Kosslyn asserts that a wide variety of psychological experiments indicate important truths concerning the nature of the format of the mental representations employed in visualizations. He also claims that neurophysiological evidence demonstrates that visualizations call upon parts of the brain that are dedicated to visual processing. Pylyshyn, by contrast, argues that the psychological evidence indicates nothing about the format of the representational media implicated in visualizations; and he denies that the neurophysiological evidence clearly possesses the significance accorded to it by Kosslyn.

---

[1] See, for example, the title of Tye 1991.

I think that it is fair to say that Kosslyn's ideas about visualization have become the orthodoxy, at least within psychology.[2] While Pylyshyn has fired some major salvos in the relatively recent past,[3] the arguments over mental imagery have therefore died down somewhat. But the issues continue to be important ones, and the formation of an orthodoxy often merely indicates consensus. There is therefore plenty of room for new ideas.

One striking shortcoming of the imagery debate is that it has been conducted without appeal to satisfactory theoretical views concerning the nature of the contents possessed by visual mental images. In particular, while appeals to content play a crucial role in Pylyshyn's responses to Kosslyn, we shall see that Pylyshyn's own ideas about the contents that are grasped during visualizations are inadequate.

I will argue, however, that we may use more refined ideas about the nature of distinctively sensory contents to vindicate many of Pylyshyn's criticisms of Kosslyn's appeals to psychological results. But I will also suggest that the fact that *distinctively sensory showing comes from subjective informativeness* contributes to an a posteriori case for thinking that some of Kosslyn's central claims about the neurophysiology of visualizations are likely to be correct.

To simplify things and to accord with most of the literature that I shall be discussing, I will concentrate exclusively upon visual mental images throughout most of this chapter. Non-visual mental imagery will be considered in the chapter's final section, however.

Some phenomenological evidence

Theoretical work on sensory mental imagery needs to be responsive to a wide range of considerations, including phenomenological ones along with data derived from experiments within psychology and neurophysiology. If we are to appreciate the bearing of distinctively sensory content upon the imagery debate, we need to have some pertinent data before us.

---

[2] As Pylyshyn recognizes: he notes, for instance, that '[o]ne of the most widely accepted claims about mental images is that they are "spatial,"', where 'the alleged spatiality of mental images is central to the claim [as made by Kosslyn] that images are *depictive* and thus unlike a language of thought [as Pylyshyn suggests they might be]' (2006, 359); see also Pylyshyn 2002a, 158.

[3] See, for example, Pylyshyn 2002a and 2006.

While the bulk of recent work on visual mental imagery has been driven by a varied range of experimental results, some of the most immediately compelling pieces of data relating to visualization are phenomenological. To quote Pylyshyn, '[i]t may well be that the most persuasive reason for believing that mental imagery involves inner perception is the subjective one: [visual mental] imagery is accompanied by an experience very similar to that of seeing'.[4]

So, visual mental images provide us with the same sort of information about visualized scenes as visual sensations provide us with concerning the scenes which we apparently see. And the *manner* in which visual mental images supply us with information about visualized scenes is bound to the phenomenological nature of vision. When we entertain visual mental images we thereby appreciate what it is like to seem to see certain sorts of scenes; and the details of any scenes that we thereby visualize are fixed by the contents of the visual appearances whose phenomenological character is thus disclosed to us by means of the relevant visual mental images.

The explicitly representational character of visualizings marks them off from visual sensations in general, however. While visualizings are like thoughts, in that they do not involve conscious deciphering of representational vehicles, they are also like thoughts in that they are episodes in which some representing evidently occurs; whereas visual sensations typically seem merely to feature encounters with the world.[5] But the representational nature of visualizings makes for a phenomenological resemblance to certain special visual episodes: namely, to those episodes in which, upon viewing pictures, we grasp the ways that the pictures show things as looking.

The phenomenological relationships between visualizings and suitable picture-viewings are reflected in many of the customary ways in which we talk about visual mental images. We naturally speak of 'viewing' visual mental images with our 'minds' eyes', for instance; indeed, we slip very easily into talk of 'picturing' things to ourselves when we visualize. Yet the idea that visualizings are importantly related to appropriate picture-viewings

---

[4] Pylyshyn 2006, 350.

[5] A recantation: Gregory 2010c—a paper whose contents are otherwise heavily drawn upon in the current chapter—wrongly conflates the fact that visualizings and thoughts lack consciously deciphered representational vehicles with the false claim that episodes of those sorts are not explicitly representational.

is somewhat puzzling. In viewing pictures, we really look at the things; but we do not literally look at the visual mental images figuring in visualizings. So what leads to our sense that visualizings are like suitable picture-viewings?

Some behavioural evidence

Phenomenological considerations make it hard to doubt that there is something especially visual about visualization and that there are also important relationships between visualizings and appropriate picture-viewings. But introspective data have often been regarded as of limited use in assessing hypotheses about the natures of the processes involved in visualization. Experimental psychologists have therefore gathered lots of other evidence. The range of relevant experiments is far too large for me to survey comprehensively here, so I shall focus upon a few striking and influential results. I will describe the sorts of results considered in this section as pieces of *behavioural* data.

Consider, to begin, the imagery scanning results that have been obtained by Kosslyn and others.[6] In a typical experiment of this type, subjects are made to produce specific visual mental images by, say, memorizing the look of a map like the one reproduced as Figure 5.1.

The subjects are instructed to focus their minds' eyes on one of the points found on the resulting visual mental image—the point on the visualized map at which a tree is marked, as it might be. They are then asked to move their focus to a different point on the visual mental image, indicating the moment at which their attention rests on the specified end point. The previous process is repeated for a range of starting points and end points.

It has been found, time and time again, that the delays between the initial focusings and the reports of the subsequent ones are proportional to the spatial distances that would lie between the counterparts of the relevant pairs of focal points found upon a faithful physical realization of what the subject has visualized. So, for example, it has been found that scanning from the tree-icon to the grass-icon on a visualized version of Figure 5.1 takes people longer than scanning from the tree-icon to the hut-icon.

---

[6] See, for example, Kosslyn 1973; see also Chapter 3 of Finke 1989 and pp. 303–10 of Pylyshyn 2006 for surveys of relevant literature and further discussion.

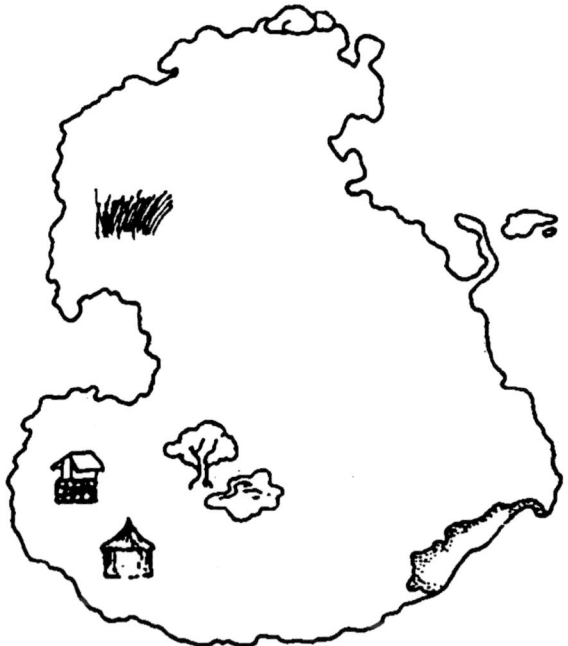

Figure 5.1. A map of a fictional island; from Kosslyn, Ball, and Reiser 1978[7]

Another well-known group of behavioural experiments, whose out-comes were first reported by Shepard and Metzler,[8] relate to 'mental rotation'. The subjects studied by Shepard and Metzler were presented with pairs of pictures of three-dimensional objects like the ones shown in Figure 5.2, where each of the pairs consisted either of representations of things having a single shape or of representations of items whose shapes were three-dimensional mirror-images of each other ('enantiomorphs').

For each of the pairs, the subjects were then instructed to use their powers of visualization in assessing whether the shapes belonging to the items shown by the pictures were the same or whether the objects were enantiomorphs. It was discovered that, for a given pair, the time taken by

---

[7] From S. M. Kosslyn, T. M. Ball, and B. J. Reiser 1978, 'Visual images preserve metric spatial information: evidence from studies of image scanning', *Journal of Experimental Psychology: Human Perception and Performance,* 4(1): 47–60, published by the American Psychological Association. Reprinted with permission.
[8] Shepard and Metzler 1971.

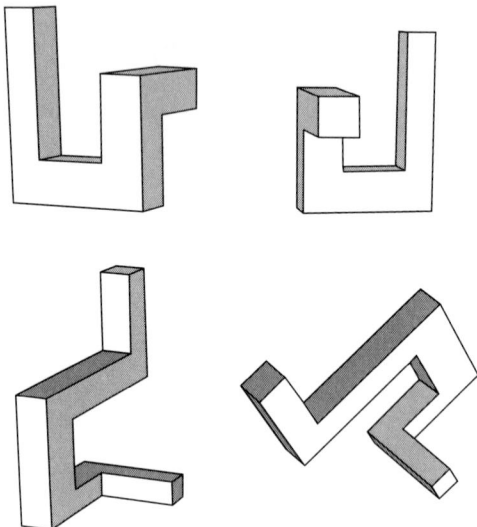

Figure 5.2. Some pairs of drawings; based on original images included in Shepard and Metzler 1971[9]

the subjects to make their assessments was proportional to the degree of angular displacement found between the represented items; intuitively, by the extent to which one would need to rotate three-dimensional realizations of the represented things if one sought to get them to line up with one another as well as possible.

A final example: the ways that things look to us in the course of real visual sensations involve non-uniform levels of visual acuity: the central regions of our visual fields provide us with much richer and more discriminating information than we get from their peripheral regions. There are standard tests which perceptual psychologists have designed to measure those variable patterns of visual resolution.

A subject may be presented with a pair of dots that are separated by a small distance, for instance. The dots may be moved around the subject's visual field, with the distance between the dots remaining constant. The subject may then be asked to indicate the points at which the dots cease to

---

[9] See R. N. Shepard and J. Metzler 1971, 'Mental rotation of three-dimensional objects', *Science* 171. Images used with permission from the American Association for the Advancement of Science.

be discriminable. By repeating that process using numerous pairs of dots that are separated by different fixed distances, and by charting the resulting responses, one can plot the ways in which the different portions of a subject's visual field resolve spatial differences to a greater or lesser degree.[10]

Finke and Kosslyn used a visualization-involving counterpart of the previous procedure to 'compare directly the fields of resolution in [visual mental] imagery and perception'.[11] They asked their subjects to gaze at pairs of real dots of the sorts described in the previous paragraph, until those subjects were able to 'form an accurate and vivid mental image of [them] and maintain the mental image indefinitely'.[12] That done, the subjects were asked to 'project'[13] one of their dot-visualizations onto a blank surface, and to visualize the movement of that pair of dots around their visual fields, where the imagined distance between the dots was to remain constant. The subjects were instructed to indicate the points at which they were unable to discriminate the visualized dots in their minds' eyes.[14] The responses were then recorded, to create a map of variations in visualizatory acuity.

Finke and Kosslyn compared the charts resulting from the two experimental processes just described. They found that 'acuity in mental imagery is reduced as objects are imagined at progressively more peripheral regions of the visual field, in the same way that acuity in perception is reduced as objects are observed at progressively more peripheral regions of the visual field'.[15]

Some neurophysiological evidence

In performing the behavioural experiments reported in the previous section, psychologists sought to gather objective measurements bearing indirectly upon the nature of the processes that occur within us when we

---

[10] Finke and Kosslyn 1980 used this procedure to provide a properly visual comparison for the imagery-based tests described in the next paragraph; see the discussion in their article from p. 128.

[11] Finke 1989, 32.

[12] Finke and Kosslyn 1980, 129.

[13] Finke and Kosslyn 1980, 129.

[14] This is a fairly rough description of the techniques employed by Finke and Kosslyn; see Finke and Kosslyn 1980, 128–30, for a more detailed description of the relevant methodology.

[15] Finke and Kosslyn 1980, 138; see pp. 130–6 for their analyses of the experimental results. The charts resulting from the visualizatory experiments are not exactly the same as the ones resulting from the experiments for genuine visual acuity; see Finke 1989, 34–5, for more discussion.

visualize. But why not address those questions more directly, by looking for links between regions of our brains and our powers of visualization?

In the course of ordinary visual experiences, light passes through our corneas, our pupils and the lenses of our eyes, before reaching our retinas. The neural signals resulting from retinal activity are carried down the optic nerves, whose fibres relay the signals to numerous parts of the brain; the preponderance of the fibres end up at the two 'lateral geniculate nuclei' in an important part of the brain known as the 'thalamus'.[16] Cell fibres from the lateral geniculate nuclei then carry messages onwards to a neural area in the cerebral cortex—the 'grey matter' that makes up the furrowed and ridged outer surfaces of our brains—known as *primary visual*, or *striate*, cortex. There are, though, various other parts of the cerebral cortex that are dedicated to vision and whose activities are ultimately dependent upon the activities of primary visual cortex; these additional visual neural areas are commonly known as *secondary visual*, or *extrastriate*, cortex.

A notable feature of some of the cerebral areas dedicated to vision is that they are *retinotopic*: adjacent parts of the relevant cortical surfaces are responsive to activity in adjacent regions of the retinal areas to which they are linked. Scans of the activity produced in retinotopic visual areas are thus like simple pictures capturing the shapes occupying portions of the visual field.[17] The resulting 'pictures' are, however, somewhat distorted, because they manifest the widespread phenomenon of 'cortical magnification'. In striate cortex, for example, '[a]bout half of the cortical surface is devoted to the central 10° of the visual field, which occupies only 1 per cent of the visual field'.[18]

Over the last couple of decades, researchers have used various types of neurological studies—ones looking at the visualizatory effects of damage to visual neural areas, for example, or ones using recently developed non-invasive methods of brain-scanning—in considering the relationships between the especially visual parts of our brains and visualizations.

---

[16] Mather 2006, 192. See pp. 192–3 of Mathers's book for a brief summary of the six sites at which the fibres of the optic nerve end, some of whose precise functions are still unknown. (The thalamus is a 'large dual-lobed mass of neurons lying in the middle of the brain at the top of the brainstem and below each cerebral cortex', and it 'relays information to the cortex from diverse brain regions' (Mather 2006, 13).)

[17] See, for example, the famous image of the flattened surface of the left side of a macaque's visual cortex initially published in Tootell et al. 1982 (as reproduced in, for example, Pylyshyn 2006, 392, and Mather 2006, 15).

[18] Mather 2006, 201.

Kosslyn, for example, reports that experimenters 'have found that the vast majority of brain areas activated during visual perception are also activated during visual mental imagery'.[19] In particular, he claims that 'when people form visual mental images of objects and "look" for details, retinotopically organized brain areas are activated in humans'.[20] Pylyshyn, however, is much more guarded: he says that, while '[t]here appears to be some evidence that mental imagery involves areas of striate cortex associated with vision',[21] most of the evidence suggests 'that only later visual areas, the [non-retinotopic] so-called visual association areas, are active in mental imagery'.[22]

Those controversies are not ones in which I am equipped to engage. But it would be disappointing if the ascription of distinctively visual contents to visual mental images—and, more generally, the ascription of distinctively sensory contents to sensory mental images—did not bear interestingly upon neurological matters. Towards the end of the chapter, I will therefore explore some ways in which views concerning distinctively sensory content may be related to questions about the neural bases for sensory mental images. In particular, I will argue that the thesis that *distinctively sensory showing comes from subjective informativeness* bears interestingly upon neurophysiological matters.

As remarked above, the most well-known recent theorists of visual mental imagery are Kosslyn and Pylyshyn. The next two sections take a closer look at some of the ideas associated with those figures.

Kosslyn's pictorialism

Kosslyn holds that episodes involving visual mental images call upon mental representations that are couched within a roughly pictorial format, one which exploits specifically visual neurological resources. More precisely, and making more explicit the conception of 'pictorial format' which Kosslyn employs, he endorses the idea that the 'representations that ultimately give rise to the experience of imagery are actual images— insofar as each part of the representation corresponds to part of the

---

[19] Kosslyn 2008, 97.

[20] Kosslyn 2008, 103, citing Kosslyn and Thompson 2003.

[21] Pylyshyn 2006, 394, who also cites some relevant references; see also Mazard et al. 2004.

[22] Pylyshyn 2006, 394, again; see the same page for a substantial list of relevant references.

represented pattern, and the distances among the representations of the parts correspond to the distances among the parts themselves'.[23]

The phenomenological flavour of episodes of visualizing may seem to lend some initial plausibility to Kosslyn's pictorialism. For it may seem natural to explain our introspective sense that visualizations are like picture-viewings by positing analogies between the processes which, in the course of visualizations and picture-viewings, underlie our appreciations of the ways that things are shown as looking. More fully, one might hold that visualizations are realized using neural occurrences which feature the deciphering of picture-like representational vehicles which are viewed by some sort of inner eye;[24] and that, in addition, our introspective sense of similarities between visualizations and picture-viewings arises from our consciousness of the various parallel steps in the processes which underlie episodes of those sorts.

The main arguments which Kosslyn originally supplied for his pictorialist approach were not phenomenological, however, but instead concerned its explanatory powers in relation to pieces of behavioural data.

Reconsider Figure 5.1. It is easy to explain why it will tend to take longer for us to scan visually from, say, the tree marked on Figure 5.1 itself to the grass marked on it than it would take for us to scan visually from the tree to the hut, given that the scans proceed at roughly the same constant rate and follow pretty direct paths. For the time taken by one's gaze to trace a fairly direct path from one point to another, at a constant speed, is proportional to the distance between the points; and the tree-icon is closer to the hut-icon than it is to the grass-icon. According to Kosslyn, a parallel line of thought provides the best explanation of the visualizatory scanning results.

---

[23] Kosslyn and Thompson 2003, 723. The notion of 'distance' employed in Kosslyn's account of a 'pictorial format', as it applies to the relationships between portions of the neural representations which are meant to encode visual mental images, is supposed by Kosslyn to be 'functional' rather than straightforwardly spatial; see, for example, Kosslyn 1981, 213–14, and p. 35 onwards of Tye 1991. This point leads to some serious worries concerning the specifically 'pictorialist' character of Kosslyn's theory (see, for instance, Pylyshyn 2006, 359–68). I have passed over those issues in the text, however. For the fundamental question upon which I want to focus is the more general one of the extent to which *any* conclusions concerning the formats of the mental representations underlying visualizations may justifiably be inferred from the experimental data commonly cited; the putatively 'pictorial' character or otherwise of the representations is really a side issue.

[24] Compare Kosslyn's idea that visualizations involve scans of picture-like representations laid out on the surface of the 'visual buffer'; see, for example, Kosslyn 1980, 6.

Kosslyn suggests that the relative distances between the points lying on a visualized version of Figure 5.1 correspond to the relative distances between the corresponding points lying on Figure 5.1 itself. He also suggests that, in performing a visualizatory scanning between two points on a visualized version of Figure 5.1, a subject will generally access at a constant rate a series of points which trace a fairly direct path between the initial point and the end point.[25] Kosslyn's explanatory strategy thus assumes that visual mental images have one of the central features which he takes to be required for their being couched in a 'pictorial format': 'the distances among the representations of the parts correspond to the distances among the parts themselves'.[26]

Consider, next, the mental rotation results. They may seem to fit very naturally with Kosslyn's pictorialism. Consider the things shown in the first pair of pictures included in Figure 5.2. Suppose that one were to assess whether or not their shapes were the same by producing, at a constant rate, a sequence of real pictures displaying the gradual rotation of the thing shown by the first picture in the pair, where the sequence ends once the shown item's orientation suitably lines up with the orientation of the object shown by the second picture in the pair. Then the amount of time taken to produce the assessment would be dependent upon the angular displacement holding between the things shown in the pair of pictures.

But now assume that Kosslyn's pictorialism is right. Assume, in particular, that one who forms a visual mental image corresponding to one of the pictures drawn from Figure 5.2 thereby produces a representation whose format is pictorial. Then a corresponding explanation of the mental rotation results relating to the pairs of pictures included in Figure 5.2 immediately suggests itself. On this explanation, the results arise because, when performing the experimental task in relation to one of the pairs of pictures, the experimental subjects produce picture-like representations at a constant rate, where those pictures display an item's gradual rotation. The lengths of the resulting sequences of inner pictures then depend upon the degree of

[25] See, for example, Kosslyn et al. 1979, 135–8 and Tye 1991, 53–6.

[26] Kosslyn and Thompson 2003, 723. Matters are in fact complicated at this point by Kosslyn's broadening of the notion of 'distance' through his introduction of the idea of a 'functional space', but (as remarked in a previous footnote) I shall ignore these complications because they are irrelevant to what follows; see, for example, Kosslyn 1981, 215–16, and Pylyshyn 2006, 259–68, for more discussion.

angular displacement holding between the things shown by the pictures in the relevant pair, yielding the observed evidence.[27]

Kosslyn holds that behavioural evidence also illuminates issues relating to the more detailed nature of the pictorial format underlying visualizations. He holds, for example, that the behavioural evidence relating to visualizatory acuity strongly suggests that 'the resolution [in the representational medium in which visual mental images are realized] is highest at the center [of the picture-like representations in that medium which realize visual mental images] . . . and decreases towards the periphery'.[28] More generally, the results indicate to Kosslyn and Finke that the 'neural mechanisms that are activated when objects are imagined at particular locations in the visual field are like those activated when objects are observed at particular locations in the visual field'.[29]

Since first developing his pictorialist position, Kosslyn has come to focus very heavily upon neurophysiological evidence, which he takes to fill out his theory by indicating how the relatively abstract psychological models of visualization which he has developed are realized within our brains.[30] Questions about possible neurological realizations of Kosslyn's models are outside the scope of the current discussion, however, so I shall now proceed to an examination of some of Pylyshyn's ideas, again focusing exclusively upon his thoughts about the behavioural data.

Pylyshyn's non-pictorialism

As we have just seen, Kosslyn holds that a large body of behavioural data is best explained using assumptions about the format of the mental representations which generate our experiences of visual mental imagery. Pylyshyn strenuously disagrees. He holds that the behavioural data can be explained merely by supposing that the 'opticality' of visual mental images derives from the nature of the contents which we grasp in visualizations, and by assuming that the processes in which the experimental subjects

---

[27] Pylyshyn writes that the mental rotation results have 'been universally interpreted as showing that images are "rotated" continuously and at constant speed in the mind and that this is, in fact, the means by which the comparison is made' (Pylyshyn 2006, 317); see also Tye 1991, 56–7.

[28] Kosslyn 1981, 214.

[29] Finke and Kosslyn 1980, 138.

[30] See Kosslyn 2008 for a helpful summary.

employ those contents are subject to various general constraints without any special connections to visual mental imagery.

Pylyshyn claims, in particular, that 'what is special about image-based thinking is that it is typically concerned with a certain sort of content or subject matter, such as optical, geometrical, or what we might call the appearance-properties of the things we are thinking about'.[31] Yet this may seem immediately to raise another question. Why should 'image-based thinking' involve *that* sort of subject matter alone, if not because of facts about the fundamentally pictorial nature of the format of the mental representations involved in visualizations?

Pylyshyn holds that visualizings are episodes in which one 'simulates' seeing something,[32] or in which one produces a simulation of what things would look like if one were to see them.[33] If he is correct, the representational restrictions noted in the previous paragraph look to be easily explicable without employing assumptions about the nature of the representational formats underlying our experiences of visual mental imagery. For our simulations of seeings will presumably be informed by our awareness of what occurs during visual episodes. Hence, on his approach, the contents involved in visualizations will naturally mirror the ways that things can look to us to be.

That last point bears significantly upon some of the behavioural data which Kosslyn adduces in support of his view. Consider, say, the scanning results. Pylyshyn holds that, when experimental subjects are asked 'to scan mentally across a visual mental image' corresponding to Figure 5.1, they take themselves to be required to 'pretend (in whatever way they can) that they are looking at [Figure 5.1] and then to use whatever knowledge they have and whatever problem-solving technique seems to them most

---

[31] Pylyshyn 2002a, 158.

[32] This is very much the dominant approach to visualization in Pylyshyn's writings; see, for example, Pylyshyn 1981, 182, 189, and 191–2, and Pylyshyn 2006, 300, 301, and 325. (Pylyshyn also speaks of 'pretendings' in this connection; see Pylyshyn 2006, 306.) It should be noted that Pylyshyn's thesis that visualizations amount to simulated seeings is not the same as the 'simulationist' view explored in Currie 1995. For Currie explicitly assumes that visual images result from the 'offline' use of portions of the post-retinal visual system, while Pylyshyn's notion of simulation is much more permissive; Pylyshyn writes, for instance, that 'the scanning experiment and many other such experiments involving mental images . . . [invite] observers to pretend (*in whatever way they can*) that they are looking at some situation' (Pylyshyn 2006, 306; emphasis added).

[33] Pylyshyn 2006, 325.

relevant, to generate the appropriate sequence of mental states'.[34] But, as just noted, our starting point in pretending to see things is likely to be our knowledge of what visual episodes involve.

In particular, we implicitly believe that if one scans visually from one point on an image to another, the duration of the scan will typically be proportional to the distance between the points. Hence our simulations of seeings will presumably reflect that fact. But now suppose that Pylyshyn is right to think that visualizations are simulated seeings. Then any experiment designed to measure the times taken 'to scan mentally between pairs of points found on a visual mental image' corresponding to, say, Figure 5.1 is likely to yield results apparently revealing that those times are proportional to the actual distances lying between the points on Figure 5.1 itself.

Pylyshyn therefore urges that 'there is no need to assume that [the scanning results arise from] any special property of the representational medium, as opposed to simply being governed by what subjects believe or infer'.[35] He takes a similar tack with regard to, say, Finke and Kosslyn's visualizatory acuity results; he claims that the visualizatory acuity data merely manifest the fact that the experimental subjects, in simulating visual sensations, drew upon their tacit knowledge of 'roughly how far into the periphery of their visual field things can be before they cease to be discriminable'.[36]

While Pylyshyn seeks to explain some of the best-known experimental results in the literature using the thesis that they arise from the 'use of tacit knowledge [by experimental subjects] to simulate aspects of real-world events, as they would appear if [the subjects] were to see them unfold',[37] it is worth noting that he does not think that all of the results can be accounted for in that fashion.

Pylyshyn expresses doubts about whether the mental rotation results can be explained along the above lines, for instance. He states that in that case 'the most likely explanation is one that appeals to the computational

---

[34] Pylyshyn 2006, 306.
[35] Pylyshyn 1981, 186. See Pylyshyn 2006, 303–10, for further discussion of the scanning results (including evidence for thinking that the results themselves are more complicated than initial appearances might suggest).
[36] Pylyshyn 2006, 312.
[37] Pylyshyn 2006, 325.

requirements of the task and to general architectural (e.g. working memory) constraints'.[38] But he notes that, even if the mental rotation results are not amenable to an explanation invoking tacit knowledge, the alternative explanation still 'applies regardless of the form of the representation'.[39] He concludes that the mental rotation results also furnish no support for Kosslyn's pictorialism.[40]

In sum, and in his own words, Pylyshyn holds that 'the phenomena and experimental findings that are cited in support of [Kosslyn's pictorialism] in fact have no bearing on the format of mental representations used, only on their content. Thus they do not provide evidence favouring one format (e.g., a picturelike format) over some other possible format (e.g., a language-like format . . .). Consequently they provide no evidence for the view that the form of representation involved when we have the experience of "seeing a mental image" is different from the form of representation involved when we have some other experience, or no experience at all.'[41]

An important general point

The disagreements between Kosslyn and Pylyshyn revolve around a range of more or less general claims.[42] It will be useful to distinguish at this juncture some of the separate points of contention.

As we saw in the previous section, Pylyshyn has employed a variety of strategies in attempting to show that numerous pieces of behavioural data do not in fact support Kosslyn's pictorialism, citing for instance the effects of tacit knowledge upon simulations of visual episodes. A lot of the back-and-forth between Kosslyn and Pylyshyn has accordingly focused upon the potential of specific non-pictorialist explanatory strategies.

Kosslyn has argued, for example, that some of the specific experimental techniques used in generating items of behavioural data militate against the use of particular non-pictorialist forms of explanation proposed by

---

[38] Pylyshyn 2006, 321.

[39] Pylyshyn 2006, 321.

[40] See Pylyshyn 2006, 316–21, for a discussion of mental rotation. More generally, see Pylyshyn 2006, 325–7, for a 'summary of some possible reasons for observed patterns of imagery findings'.

[41] Pylyshyn 2006, 287.

[42] See Pylyshyn 2002b for a helpful discussion of five separate strands in the above debates, including some which I will not explicitly consider in what follows.

Pylyshyn;[43] while Pylyshyn has developed experiments whose results are supposedly explicable using his non-pictorialist approach, and which he holds to sit much less happily with Kosslyn's pictorialist position.[44] But those relatively narrow debates seem clearly to be manifestations of a more general and fundamental disagreement between Kosslyn and Pylyshyn, one whose substance can be appreciated without a refined grasp of experimental methodologies.

A lot of behavioural data indicates that our performance in visualization tasks is similar to our performance in tasks in which we really see things, and indeed in which we comprehendingly view pictures. Kosslyn holds that the relevant results should be explained using hypotheses relating to the natures of the mental processes which underlie visualizations. In particular, he thinks that the results should be explained using suppositions pertaining to the format of the mental representations figuring in those processes. He therefore takes the scanning experiments, say, to serve as a 'window on the mind'[45]—as indirectly revealing what goes on within our brains during visualizations.

But one might well wonder how the behavioural evidence could immediately support the conclusions which Kosslyn takes it to support. For our performance in the relevant visualization tasks seems to be dictated in the first instance by our grasp of the *contents* which we entertain when visualizing, rather than by facts about *the nature of the representational media* which supply the vehicles for those contents. It is perhaps this very simple thought which has driven many of Pylyshyn's attempts to rebut Kosslyn's claims to have found behavioural support for his pictorialist theorizing. That straightforward idea is certainly suggested by the quotation from Pylyshyn which concluded the previous section, for instance.

The arguments between Kosslyn and Pylyshyn thus point up a very general issue concerning the proper morals which may be drawn from the behavioural data concerning visualization. But that issue—one which relates to the explanatory roles of assumptions concerning the format of

---

[43] See, for example, Kosslyn's brief discussion of an experiment testing for the presence of an 'oblique effect' in visualization (1981, 239), where the relatively recondite nature of the pertinent visual phenomenon is meant to block the use of a non-pictorialist explanation which invokes tacit knowledge.

[44] See, for instance, the discussion in pp. 193–9 of Pylyshyn 1981, which describes some variants on Kosslyn's scanning experiments.

[45] Denis and Kosslyn 1999.

visual mental images as opposed to ones concerning their contents—will evidently be hard to resolve unless we have a decent account of the nature of the contents which we grasp during visualizations. Do Pylyshyn's own suggestions provide us with an adequate account of those contents?

More on Pylyshyn

As we have seen, Pylyshyn calls on a couple of claims about what visualizations involve. He sometimes assumes that one who visualizes a scene simulates seeing the scene. And he sometimes takes it that one who visualizes a scene simulates how things would look to him if he were to see the scene. Each of those accounts evidently connects the contents which are grasped during visualizations to sight. But the putative connections are weaker than they need to be.

Imagine a blind person who possesses an impressive fund of factual knowledge about vision; she is, for example, highly knowledgeable about how long various sorts of visual processes take and about the patterns of visual acuity found in normal vision.

The person may be able to simulate seeing a certain sort of scene, or to simulate how some scene would look to her, merely by performing theoretical reasoning using her factual knowledge about vision. She may engage, for example, in an elaborate imagining of what a scene looks like to her, just by entertaining verbal descriptions of what she supposedly sees ('It's a bright day, bright enough to make me squint a bit. I can see two young girls. One of them has long hair and is wearing trousers . . . '). And, in so doing, she may use her knowledge about vision to derive highly plausible-sounding conclusions about the properties of the visual episodes which she is pretending to undergo.

But suppose that the person's simulations—and indeed all of the rest of her life—contain nothing which could apprise her of what it is like to see things. Perhaps her imaginative episodes are sometimes accompanied by hearings of sounds with her 'inner ear', for instance, which could apprise her of what it is like to hear things which she is not then hearing. And perhaps they sometimes incorporate wholly 'inner' counterparts of tactile sensations, ones which could apprise her of what it would be like to have tactile sensations which she is not then having. But assume that, by contrast, the envisaged blind person simply has no 'inner eye': neither

her actual sensations nor any purely inner counterparts thereof acquaint her with what it is like to see things.

Then the envisaged blind person's simulated seeings, and her simulations of how things would look to her if she were to see them, surely do not amount to visualizings. For visual mental images are representations which *show* things as looking certain ways. And, as emphasized in Chapter 3, the visual form of distinctively sensory showing figuring in visualizations—showing things as *looking* certain ways—flows from the way in which visualizations may apprise us of what it is like to have visual sensations of appropriate sorts. The especially visual nature of visualizations thus derives, at least in part, from the fact that our ability to visualize things is bound to our ability to appreciate what it is like to have visual sensations.

Pylyshyn's position ignores that fact: recall his statement that the scanning experiments invite subjects to 'pretend (*in whatever way they can*) . . . to generate the appropriate sequence of mental states'.[46] More generally, Pylyshyn's claim that the special nature of 'image-based thinking' flows from its concern with 'a certain sort of content or subject matter, such as optical, geometrical, or what we might call the appearance-properties of the things we are thinking about'[47] is too weak. For it overlooks the peculiarly visual way in which visual mental images present to us their 'optical' subject matters.

As we have just seen, Pylyshyn's content-based account of the especially visual nature of visualizations is inadequate. But the theory of distinctively sensory content presented in Chapter 3 provides an obvious alternative approach, one that nonetheless concentrates solely upon the nature of the contents belonging to visual mental images. Can the idea that visual mental images possess distinctively visual contents be used in accounting for any of the pieces of phenomenological and behavioural evidence assembled earlier?

Revisiting the phenomenological data

The thesis that visual mental images have distinctively visual contents easily sidesteps the problems outlined at the end of the previous section for Pylyshyn's account of the contents which we grasp during visualizations.

---

[46] Pylyshyn 2006, 306; emphasis added.   [47] Pylyshyn 2002a, 158.

Distinctively sensory showing comes from subjective informativeness. Hence, one who entertains a visual mental image thereby appreciates what it is like to have a sensation in which things look the way that the image shows things as looking. The ascription of distinctively visual contents to visual mental images thus rightly implies that our powers of visualization are indissolubly linked to our ability to appreciate what it is like to see things. More generally, the claim that visual mental images have distinctively visual contents makes good sense of plenty of pieces of phenomenological data relating to visualization.

Visualize a table. Your ability to obey that instruction is bound to your general ability to appreciate what it is like to see things, as just noted. More specifically, however, your capacity to visualize the particular type of table displayed by your visual mental image is bound to your ability to appreciate what it is like to seem to see the specific kind of table displayed by your visual mental image. That second, narrower, phenomenological point is again easily handled by applying this book's theory of distinctively sensory content to your visual mental image.

For *scene-showing corresponds to seeming*: the nature of the table which you visualized corresponds to the nature of the table which would be seen by anyone to whom things looked the way that your visual mental image showed things as looking. Yet the subjective informativeness of distinctively sensory contents means that your ability to produce a visual mental image which showed things as looking a certain way is bound to your ability to appreciate what it is like to have a visual sensation in which things look that way. Hence your ability to visualize the sort of table which you visualized was bound to your ability to appreciate what it is like to seem to see a table of the particular kind which you visualized.

An important phenomenological difference between visualizations and visual sensations in general was noted above: visualizations are explicitly representational episodes, whereas visual sensations typically are not. That observation may be addressed merely by noting that visualizations involve graspings of distinctively visual contents. Visualizations are therefore representational in a way that real visual sensations—which, as noted earlier, generally seem merely to involve encounters with the world, rather than expressions of content—usually are not. Yet this representational aspect of visualizations makes them resemble those visual episodes in which we grasp the ways that pictures show things as looking, even though visualizations are unlike picture-viewings in that the former do not them-selves feature relevant uses of our eyes.

The idea that visual mental images are like pictures which show how things look, in having distinctively visual contents, thus enables us to understand some of the most notable phenomenological features of visu-alizations. My own conjecture is that all of the phenomenological rela-tionships holding between visualizations, real visual sensations, and suitable picture-viewings can be accounted for using the preceding thesis. But that is merely a conjecture. What remains to be found, however, are any aspects of the phenomenology of visualization which are explicable only once one invokes the sorts of claims about representational format that constitute Kosslyn's pictorialist approach to visual mental images.

In the light of the concerns which have most openly driven the imagery debate, however, the interest of all those points is somewhat limited. Kosslyn's pictorialism is not founded upon phenomenological consider-ations, after all. How, then, does the view that visual mental images have distinctively visual contents bear upon the behavioural data?

Revisiting the behavioural data

It is easy to share Pylyshyn's unease at the way in which, say, the scanning results have led researchers to conclusions about the pictorial format of the mental representations involved in generating visual mental imagery. For a subject's performance on a scanning task does seem to be most immedi-ately explicable by the nature of the contents which he grasps during the resulting episodes of visualization, rather than by facts about the represen-tational media that his brain uses throughout the task. This can be illus-trated by considering an elaboration of some intuitive ideas concerning the scanning results.

Suppose that you perform a typical scanning task. Then having, say, memorized Figure 5.1, you will produce a visual mental image which focuses on the proposed starting point. Next, you will 'scan' from that initial point to the specified end point. That is, you will produce, at a constant rate, a series of visual mental images whose shifting points of focus lead in a relatively direct manner from the starting point to the specified end point. But the length of that series of visual mental images will reflect the distance lying between the two relevant points on Figure 5.1 itself.

The amount of time which it will take for you to scan from the starting point to the end point will thus correspond to the distance separating those two points on the map itself.

One might think that the measurements obtained in the course of standard scanning experiments are owed to the fact that the experimental subjects performed the relevant scanning tasks in the way just described. Can that thought be reinforced without introducing assumptions about the format of the mental representations that are involved in generating visual mental images?

Suppose that some subject, having memorized the look of Figure 5.1, is asked to perform a scanning task. The subject will initially produce a visual mental image which shows things as looking a certain way, where that way for things to look has the relevant starting point as its focus. The subject will then produce, at a constant rate, a series of further visual mental images. And the ways that those additional visual mental images show things as looking will involve a sequence of focal points which trace a relatively direct path from the starting point to the specified end point. But all that implies that the time taken by the subject to perform the scanning task will be proportional to the distance lying between the starting point and the end point on Figure 5.1 itself.

By adopting the explanatory model outlined in the previous paragraph, then, we may explain any scanning results that are obtained in relation to Figure 5.1. More generally, we may adapt that explanatory model to other cases, thereby covering other bodies of scanning results. Yet the explanatory model, while it sticks very closely to some appealingly simple ideas about the processes by means of which people perform scanning tasks, does not call upon Kosslyn's pictorialism. Instead, it merely invokes claims about the ways that some visual mental images show things as looking, along with an auxiliary assumption about the rate at which the visual mental images are produced.

Appropriate uses of theoretical ideas about distinctively visual content also let us stick closely to very natural explanations of the mental rotation results. Suppose, for instance, that a subject is presented with one of the pairs of drawings reproduced in Figure 5.2, where the subject is set the task of assessing whether the shapes of the items shown are identical or whether they are enantiomorphs.

Assume that, in performing the task, the subject starts by producing a visual mental image which shows something as looking a certain way, where one of the drawings in the relevant pair also shows things as looking that same way. Suppose that the subject then produces, at a constant rate, a sequence of visual mental images, where the ways that those subsequent visual mental images show things as looking feature the apparent rotation of a single item. And assume that the process continues until the subject reaches a visual mental image which settles immediately whether the item figuring in the way that the visual mental image shows things as looking has the same shape as the shape of the thing shown in the remaining drawing.

Then the length of the resulting sequence of images will depend upon the degree of angular displacement holding between the items shown in the original drawings. But, given the constant rate at which the visual mental images were produced along with the smoothness of the rotation which they involved, the length of time required for the subject to perform the experimental task will likewise be proportional to the relevant degree of angular displacement, as initially observed by Shepard and Metzler.

It is worth noting that some of the finer details of this book's theory of distinctively sensory content allow us to make sense of features of the explanatory models just sketched which might otherwise seem mysterious. So, for example, the mooted explanations of the scanning results assumed that the ways which visual mental images show things as looking can involve 'focal points'. And that assumption might seem to invite the introduction of an 'inner eye' which scans representations whose format is pictorial, and which focuses on portions of those inner pictures—reintroducing Kosslyn's pictorialism by the back door.

But reconsider the map reproduced as Figure 5.1. Produce a visual mental image which 'focuses' upon, say, the house-icon. Each possible visual sensation in which things look the way that your visual mental image shows things as looking will have a certain subjective character. In particular, any possible visual sensation with that subjective character will thereby be one in which the viewer's visual focus is aimed at a certain sort of apparent thing. In that sense, then, the very way that your visual mental image shows things as looking involves a specific point of visual focus. This is just a matter of the nature of the image's distinctively visual content, however, and it does not force us to start seriously bandying about talk of 'inner eyes'.

In sum, the claim that visual mental images have distinctively visual contents allows us to explain the facts about response times that have been logged in the scanning and mental rotation experiments, and to do so in a manner which is faithful to our most natural thoughts about why those results obtain. But the explanations respect Pylyshyn's important general insight about the limitations of the behavioural data bearing on visualization; they bear out his belief that some of 'what is special about imaginal thinking might simply be the fact that mental imagery is associated with certain contents . . . [rather than] the way the information is encoded'.[48] For the explanations—and the analogous ones which are available for a host of further well-known behavioural results pertaining to visualization—never advert to features of the representational media deployed by our brains in the course of producing our experiences of visual mental images; they restrict themselves to claims about the nature of the contents the images possess.

Visualizatory acuity

The behavioural explanations formulated in the previous section are appealing ones, I think. But there are important questions about the detailed natures of processes of visualization which the explanations do not themselves address.

Why, for example, do the visualizations produced in response to scanning tasks tend to take the form described in the previous section? Is that form—for example, the spatially sequential nature of the ways for things to look that figure in the contents of the visual mental images prompted by scanning tasks—indicative of 'properties and mechanisms [which] are *intrinsic* or *constitutive* of having and using mental images'?[49] Or is it rather determined by, say, 'the nature of thinking in general, together with our tacit knowledge of the situation being imagined, how this knowledge is organized, and how we interpret the imagining task'?[50]

Those particular questions are not ones for which I have any answers. There are some bits of behavioural data in relation to which parallel questions seem to be particularly pressing, however. More specifically, reconsider the visualizatory acuity results described towards the outset of this chapter. Those results belong to a family of pieces of data which suggest that visualizations are constrained in ways that reflect anatomically

[48] Pylyshyn 2006, 289.   [49] Pylyshyn 2006, 289.   [50] Pylyshyn 2006, 289.

derived bounds upon human vision.[51] Are those constraints upon visual-izations themselves direct corollaries of the physiology of the human visual system?

As we have seen already, Pylyshyn suggests that the visualizatory acuity results flow from the ways in which the performance of experimental subjects is shaped by their tacit knowledge about vision, and in particular their awareness of 'roughly how far into the periphery of their visual field things can be before they cease to be discriminable'.[52] Kosslyn and Finke hold, by contrast, that the results are owed to relationships between the neural bases for visualizations and for vision proper.[53] How does the idea that visual mental images have distinctively visual contents fit into these disagreements?

Let's begin by considering the very idea of a visual mental image's having varying resolution. Kosslyn and Finke regard variations in visuali-zatory acuity as deriving from certain corresponding variations in the properly visual neural bases of visualizations. But their approach does not identify the nature of visualizatory acuity as it presents itself to us in our conscious lives; it does not isolate those distinctive aspects of our conscious experiences of visualizing which make it natural to claim that there are varying levels of resolution within visual mental images.

Think about the real visual case. The varying levels of resolution that are manifested by our visual sensations amount to variations of certain sorts in the ways that things look to us. In particular, the facts apparently made manifest to us by the more peripheral parts of our visual fields are, in certain respects, less discriminating than those apparently captured by the more central parts. The varying levels of resolution which seem to be displayed by visual mental images are similar: there is a distinction between the more and less peripheral portions of the ways that visual mental images show things as looking; and the acuity results suggest that the more peripheral regions of the ways that visual mental images show things as looking make fewer discriminations than the less peripheral regions.

We can use the idea that visual mental images have distinctively visual contents to elaborate nicely that initial account of what it is for a visual

---

[51] See the 'imaging to the point of overflow' results briefly described on pp. 138–40 of Kosslyn et al. 1979 for more data of the above type.
[52] Pylyshyn 2006, 312.
[53] Finke and Kosslyn 1980, 138.

mental image to have variable resolution. Suppose that some visual mental image's distinctively visual content characterizes a certain visual sensation-type as being a way that things look, whether in the course of a visual sensation or from a perspective. And suppose that, in addition, any possible sensation of the relevant type involves the instantiation of a certain pattern of varying degrees of visual resolution across the parts of the subject's visual field. Then the way that the visual mental image shows things as looking—and hence the very distinctively visual content which we grasp in entertaining the image—will thereby also involve that shared pattern of variable levels of resolution.

The pattern of resolutions which belongs to a visual mental image thus corresponds to the common pattern of resolutions instantiated by those visual sensations in which things look as the image shows them as looking. The visualizatory acuity results therefore suggest the following. Suppose that one performs a visualization, thereby grasping a certain distinctively visual content which identifies some visual sensation-type in terms of what it is like to have visual sensations in which things look that way. Then the visual sensations of that type will involve a common pattern of visual resolutions, one that approximates the pattern of visual resolutions that is instantiated by the visual sensations which we actually have.

What is responsible for that approximation? The mere idea that visual mental images have distinctively sensory contents does not suggest an answer to that question. One might think, to adapt Pylyshyn's ideas, that the acuity results merely reflect ways in which our tacit knowledge of what seeing is really like somehow places restrictions on the range of distinctively visual contents which we come to grasp through visualizations. In the absence of some fuller account of why our tacit knowledge should have that effect, however, it is worth noting the availability of another approach, one which is perhaps more natural and which effectively adapts to the current context the stance taken by Kosslyn and Finke.

The variations in visual acuity across regions of our visual fields correlate, initially, with retinal differences: the region of highest visual acuity corresponds to the fovea, a physiologically very distinctive region of the retina, and the increasing loss of visual acuity away from that most acute region corresponds to an increasing alteration in certain physiological features. Those retinal differences also correlate with subsequent cortical ones. For, as noted already in this chapter, some of the neural areas devoted to vision amount to distorted retinotopic maps of portions of the visual field. But the distortions present in those maps seem to correspond nicely to acuity differences. More acute regions of the visual field appear to map onto larger areas of the striate visual cortex than those less acute regions of the visual field which are nonetheless the same size, for example.[54]

Faced by all that, one might well wonder whether the visualizatory acuity results somehow derive from the neurological circumstances, which seem to reflect the variations in visual acuity across our real visual fields. One might wonder, for example, whether the cortical magnification exhibited by the retinotopic map lying across the surface of the striate visual cortex is not partly responsible for the visualizatory acuity results; or whether the work is not at least done by some later visual areas of the brain, ones whose organization reflects in some relevant way the cortical magnification occurring across the striate visual cortex and in other visual regions of our brains.

On the suggested approach, then, the nature of visual neural areas somehow constrains the nature of the distinctively visual contents which belong to the visual mental images which we produce. More specifically, the view holds that the neural correlates of facts about real visual acuity somehow restrict the patterns of visual resolutions featuring in the visual sensation-types contained in the distinctively visual contents belonging to our visual mental images. But are there any independent reasons for think-ing that visual neural areas might play a significant role in shaping facts about the distinctively visual contents which we grasp during visualizations? The next section will address that question, by arguing that the thesis that *distinctively sensory showing comes from subjective informativeness* may form part of a strong a posteriori case for answering the question affirmatively.

Neurophysiology and subjective informativeness

Here is a very general form of reasoning, one which has—to put it with maximum pretension—a 'transcendental' shape.

Suppose that we are given a type R of representations, one of whose characteristics is the possession of contents of a certain sort—*S-contents*, let's say—by its instances. And suppose that the conditions in which we come to grasp the contents of the relevant representations are subject to a range of

---

[54] See, for example, Cowey and Rolls 1974; plus Duncan and Boynton 2003.

general constraints—the *R-interpretative conditions*, for short.[55] Then we may be able to establish interesting conclusions about *R*-representations, by thinking about the ways in which it is possible—practically possible or metaphysically possible or . . . —for us to grasp *S*-contents while being subject to the *R*-interpretative conditions.

Chapter 6 will apply that strategy in examining how pictures may express distinctively visual contents. Can it also be applied to shed light upon questions about how visual mental images come to possess their distinctively visual contents?

Visualizations are like many picture-viewings, in that they issue in our grasp of distinctively visual contents. But the ways in which we get at the distinctively visual contents of visual mental images and pictures are nonetheless very different; that is, to employ the schematic framework developed two paragraphs back, the *R*-interpretative conditions with which visual mental images are associated are very different to the *R*-interpretative conditions associated with those pictures that are distinctively visual representations. Most obviously, picture-viewings revolve around proximate uses of our eyes, whereas visualizations do not. Visualizations are, then, wholly internal episodes which nonetheless—by virtue of the fact that *distinctively sensory showing comes from subjective informativeness*—lead us to an awareness of what it is like to have visual sensations in which things look certain ways. How are such episodes possible?

Certain suppositions about broad features of the relevant mechanisms seem plausible in the light of some trends discernible in current thinking about the relationships between the visual brain and visual consciousness. The subjective characters of real visual sensations presumably somehow derive, at least in large measure, from neurological events which occur

---

[55] Given a type *R* of representations, a theory of the nature of *S*-contents, along with an appropriate identification of the *R*-interpretative conditions, may suggest a reductive account of what it is to be an *R*-representation: the *R*-representations are simply those representations which possess *S*-contents and which are subject to the *R*-interpretative constraints. So, for example, it might be claimed that the pictures that depict things are merely those distinctively visual representations which are subject to certain broad hermeneutic conditions; or it might be held that what it is for someone to entertain a visual mental image is for the person to undergo a suitable wholly internal episode which results in the person's coming to grasp a distinctively visual content. I do not think that the preceding reductive approach to depictive pictures works, because I think that there are depictive pictures that do not show things as looking certain ways (see Chapter 6); but I am less sure about what to say concerning the corresponding reductive approach to visualizations (although it is not assumed anywhere in this book).

within visual neural areas in response to retinal stimulations. So one might hazard that wholly internal episodes in which we come to be aware of the subjective characters of visual sensations feature non-retinally stimulated activity in the visual parts of our brains, activity which overlaps what would have occurred in those neural areas if we had really enjoyed visual sensations having the relevant subjective characters.[56]

The conjectures in the last paragraph thus suggest that any episode in which one grasps a distinctively visual content, in the absence of suitable prompting visual sensations, will nonetheless have to involve activity in neural visual areas. More precisely, they suggest that any wholly internal episode in which one grasps a distinctively visual content that involves a certain way for things to look will be accompanied by the activation of, at least, any visual neural areas whose activity is a correlate of the subject's awareness of what it is like for things to look that way in the course of a visual episode. And there is a lot of evidence that indicates that episodes involving visual mental images are indeed accompanied by visual neuro-logical activity, even though, as noted previously in this chapter, there is disagreement over the precise force of the data.[57]

The fact that *distinctively sensory showing comes from subjective informativeness* thus promises to build a bridge from theses about the visual nature of the *contents* which are grasped during visualizations to theses about the visual nature of the *neural mechanisms* which our brains exploit during those episodes. For the subjectively informative ways in which visual sensa-tion-types are identified by distinctively visual contents may require that

---

[56] Tononi and Koch (2008, 248) cite evidence which suggests that, while activity in the primary visual cortex is relevant to visual attention, it does not fix the subjective character of our visual sensations themselves. If that is right (and see Zeki and Bartels 1999 for some data which might indicate that it isn't), and given the supposition in the text, it may therefore be that only activity in later visual areas is required for us to be aware of the subjective characters of visual sensations. The idea that the involvement of visual parts of the brain in visualizations reflects the subjectively informative nature of distinctively visual contents therefore does not immediately force us towards the controversial view that early visual areas must be activated during visualizations.

[57] A lot of the experimental evidence relating to visualization revolves around imaginative activities. Visual memories are, however, another important range of episodes that involve visual mental imagery—and therefore, on the current approach, graspings of distinctively visual contents. See, for instance, Damasio et al. 1993 and Le Bihan et al. 1993 for evidence that visual rememberings activate properly visual areas of the brain; Handy et al. (2004, 632) state, with accompanying references, that 'the emerging consensus is that the retrieval of visual representations from memory leads to the reactivation of cortical areas that were initially activated during the perceptual encoding of those representations'.

those parts of our brains which enable us to enjoy genuine visual sensations must also play a role in visualizations. While the distinctively visual nature of the contents which figure in visualizations may be what explains why visual mental images are significantly visual in one important sense, the very distinctively visual nature of those contents may mean that visualizations are visual in other important senses as well.[58]

Non-visual mental imagery

The previous discussions focused upon visual mental imagery. I shall therefore conclude the current chapter by briefly broadening its perspective, to take in non-visual sensory mental imagery.

Consider the auditory analogues of visualizations, in which we produce auditory mental images which show things as sounding certain ways from perspectives or in the course of auditory sensations. Let's call those episodes *inner hearings*. Treating inner hearings as episodes in which we grasp distinctively auditory contents enables us to understand some of the immediately apparent phenomenological relationships between inner hearings and outer ones.

The information which is provided to us by inner hearings is, for instance, bound to the phenomenological character of hearing proper. And the ascription of distinctively auditory contents to auditory mental images respects that fact, for reasons that are parallel to ones that we rehearsed in the visual case. The fact that *distinctively sensory showing comes from subjective*

---

[58] According to the view mooted in the text, the subjectively informative nature of the distinctively visual contents which we grasp during visualizations means that visualizations will have to involve appropriate visual neural areas. It should be noted, though, that the proposed position apparently leaves open the precise amount of further explanatory weight that is to be borne by the assumption that visual parts of the brain are involved in visualizations, because it only posits a fairly specific role for visual parts of the brain in relation to visualization. So, assuming the view stated in the text, it might be that the acuity results for visual imagery are best explained by the involvement of visual neural areas in visualizations, and in particular by the fact that relevant retinotopic visual neural areas exhibit cortical magnification. Yet, again assuming that view, it might also be that Pylyshyn is correct in holding that the best explanations of many other pieces of experimental data (like, for instance, facts concerning how people perform in the 'additive colour mixing' tasks discussed on pp. 297–9 of Pylyshyn 2006) involve the assumption that the performances of the experimental subjects are guided by their tacit beliefs concerning visual matters. (Kosslyn (1981, 229) acknowledges that tacit beliefs probably play a central role in the colour-mixing tasks.) (Many thanks to an anonymous referee for *Mind and Language* for raising these issues.)

informativeness implies, for example, that one who entertains an auditory mental image therefore appreciates what it is like to have an auditory sensation in which things sound the way that the image shows them as sounding. And it also implies that the details of any scene that is shown by the auditory mental image derive entirely from those auditory appearances whose subjective characters are disclosed to the person by the auditory mental image that he has entertained.

But the representational character of inner hearings means that they are, in that respect, very different from outer hearings in general; for the latter typically seem merely to involve encounters with the world. It does mean, though, that inner hearings are somewhat similar to a restricted range of hearings—namely, those in which we listen comprehendingly to those playbacks of audio recordings which amount to distinctively auditory representations. Yet that last resemblance does not force us towards an auditory analogue of Kosslyn's pictorialism. For we may cater for the resemblance merely by noting that comprehending hearings of suitable playbacks are like inner hearings in that episodes of both sorts result in our grasping distinctively auditory contents.

Despite the previous resemblance between inner hearings and comprehending hearings of suitable playbacks, there is one major way in which they differ: inner hearings are wholly internal episodes. The distinctively auditory contents belonging to auditory mental images are nonetheless subjectively informative. Hence we can pose an analogue of the 'transcendental' question explored in the previous section: how could we grasp distinctively auditory contents during wholly internal episodes, given that those episodes must issue in an appreciation of what it is like to have auditory sensations in which things sound certain ways?

Again, it seems plausible that auditory neural areas will need to be activated during any wholly internal episodes which carry us to an appreciation of the phenomenological characters of auditory sensations. The distinctively auditory nature of the contents which we grasp during inner hearings—in particular the fact that *distinctively sensory showing comes from subjective informativeness*—thus suggests that properly auditory parts of our brains must play active roles in those episodes, a suggestion which chimes with some relevant neurological data.[59]

---

[59] See, for example, Bunzeck et al. 2005, Kraemer et al. 2005, and Zatorre and Halpern 2005 for discussion of the neural correlates of auditory mental imagery.

To conclude: the theory of distinctively sensory content developed previously has the resources to lead us to a better understanding of sensory mental imagery, by helping us to appreciate the sources of felt similarities between real sensations and corresponding kinds of episodes in which we entertain sensory mental images. It can also help us to chart more precisely the proper roles for assumptions concerning the formats of the mental representations which underlie episodes involving sensory mental images. And it may enable us to connect the distinctively sensory nature of the contents which sensory mental images possess to the sensory nature of the neurological mechanisms which seem to be implicated in their production.

6

Pictures

Most people, if asked to voice their first thoughts about what makes an item a picture of something, would gesture at facts that are supposedly manifested in the ways that pictures look to us; at the fact that pictures 'resemble' their objects with regard to their shapes and colours, for instance, or at the fact that pictures 'look like' what they show. Our sense that pictures are visual in special ways thus has a lot to do with the special relationships which we take to obtain between the contents which pictures possess and the ways in which pictures make their contents available to us.

Indeed, philosophers have sometimes talked as though the particularly visual nature of picturing resides solely on the special relationships just remarked. So, Walton says that 'there is something especially visual about pictorial representation'. But, as he notes, the especially visual nature of pictures cannot rest merely in the fact that pictures are to be looked at, for 'so are written words, and we use our eyes on graphs and diagrams as well'. He then states that what is especially visual about pictures 'lies in the particular nature of the visual experiences that pictures provide'.[1]

Similarly, Lopes asks '[w]hat . . . it mean[s] to say that a picture shows how O looks, when seeing O in the picture is not just like seeing O face to face'. His question is very naturally construed as relating to the nature of the contents which pictures possess: our talk of what a picture 'shows us' sounds analogous to our talk about what a passage of text 'tells us', and in the latter case we are signalling putative facts about content. But Lopes passes over that reading of his question, seeking to answer it using observations concerning how our understandings of pictures are shaped by the ways that pictures themselves look to us; he states that '[t]he answer lies in

---

[1] That quotation and the preceding ones are from Walton 2008, 118.

the principle that seeing an object in a picture depends upon and expresses knowledge of the object's appearance'.[2]

Those quotations nicely illustrate how philosophical work on pictorial representation has been apt to neglect the crucial distinction between theorizing about the contents of pictures and theorizing about how it is that we are able to grasp the contents of pictures.[3] While pictures doubtless may express their contents to us in especially visual ways, though, their special visualness does not always rest upon that fact alone. For the contents of many pictures are peculiarly visual, a fact which is reflected by our talk of the pictures as 'showing what things look like'.

Recent philosophical theories of picturing have not generally been theories of content, then. They have instead tended to be 'analyses of depiction', to use a phrase explained in the next section of this chapter. Later parts of this chapter will argue that the recent focus upon depiction has led to an oversimplified conception of the aims that should guide philosophical theorizing about pictorial representation. The chapter's later sections will also provide additional elaborations of the thought, first explored in the previous chapter's discussion of the neural bases for sensory mental imagery, that the subjective informativeness of distinctively sensory contents has important implications for how distinctively sensory contents may be expressed using media of different sorts.

---

[2] That quotation and the preceding one are from Lopes 2005, 46.

[3] Part II of Kulvicki 2006, which is inspired by Haugeland's paper on 'Representational Genera' (see Haugeland 1998, 171–206), includes some relatively detailed theorizing about the contents of pictures. The approach to pictorial contents which Kulvicki advocates is very counter-intuitive, however: he restricts the core contents of pictures in such a way that the core content of a picture only features visual information which is involved in our experience of viewing the picture itself. (Kulvicki's view consequently implies, for example, that the fundamental contents of ordinary photographs do not settle whether the pictures represent scenes laid out in depth or merely flat marked surfaces that are like the pictures themselves (Kulvicki 2006, 167).) Blumson (2010) also formulates a theory of pictorial contents, using standard ideas drawn from possible world semantics, but his theory is too general to capture most of what is interesting about the contents of pictures. His account—which treats the contents of pictures as analogous to the contents of indexical sentences of natural languages— does nothing to explain why, for example, a picture which shows things as looking certain ways, and thus depicts a horse, is able thereby only to represent visible features of the depicted horse; his theory also does nothing to cater for, say, the ways in which our grasps of the contents of pictures are able to underwrite visual recognitional capacities and the like, because his account contains nothing which reflects the distinctiveness of the 'showing' performed by those pictures that show things as looking certain ways.

Analyses of depiction

Many writers have remarked that pictures are involved in a wide range of representational relationships.[4] A suitable picture of a ragged man in irons may well be a symbol of 'the unregenerated human soul held in bondage by its natural desires', for instance. But that aspect of the picture's significance is evidently built upon more primitive layers of content, ones which are more especially pictorial.[5] To use a term generally adopted in the recent philosophical literature on pictorial representation, the items which a picture represents on account of the properly pictorial layers of its content—a ragged man in irons, as it might be, rather than the human soul's continuing enslavement to its base needs—are the things which the picture *depicts*.

The introduction to a recent anthology of philosophical papers on pictures states that '[p]hilosophical accounts of depiction aim, first and foremost, to answer the metaphysical question of what it is for one thing to depict another. That is, they aim to provide individually necessary and jointly sufficient conditions for being a picture of some object.'[6] In line with that quotation, numerous philosophers have sought to identify 'individually necessary and jointly sufficient conditions' for being a picture which depicts a so-and-so. The resulting *analyses of depiction* are meant to identify the exact conditions under which something counts as a picture which represents a so-and-so in a properly pictorial manner. Abell, Budd, Hopkins, Peacocke, and Wollheim all offer analyses of depiction, for example.[7] I'll say that an analysis of depiction is *correct* just in case the

---

[4] See, for instance, Walton 1974, 350–1; Schier 1986, 1–2; Peacocke 1987, 383; Budd 1993, 155 and 172; Hopkins 1995, 425 and 1998, 6–9; and Abell 2009, 183.

[5] See Panofsky [1939] 1972, 194, for the quotation. (Panofsky is perfectly aware of the sorts of dependency relationships cited in the text; see, for instance, Panofsky [1939] 1972, 3–17.)

[6] Abell and Bantinaki 2010, 2.

[7] Abell 2009, 217. Budd (1993) does not explicitly state his view as involving an 'iff', although he says that '[t]he primary task of a theory of depiction is the characterization of what it is to be a picture', and he means to offer a theory of depiction; so his account clearly is meant to identify necessary and sufficient conditions. Hopkins presents his theory using an 'iff' (see, for example, Hopkins 1998, 77), as does Peacocke (1987, 388). Finally, see Wollheim 2003, 5 (although Wollheim speaks of 'representation' rather than 'depiction'). In a different vein, Kulvicki offers some conditions that are meant to be 'necessary and sufficient for a representational system to be pictorial', which he takes to result in a 'theory of depiction' (both quotations from Kulvicki 2006, 63). But the resulting notions of 'depiction' and 'pictorialness' are evidently meant to be fruitful theoretical generalizations of more

conditions that it incorporates are indeed individually necessary and jointly sufficient for being a picture which depicts a so-and-so.

The category of representational pictures is very diverse. It encompasses pictures that differ enormously from one another in apparently fundamental ways. To take some cases bound to a relatively short period in the West's history, for instance, the illustrations in Anglo-Saxon manuscripts generally differ strikingly from paintings from the High Renaissance, both of which differ notably in turn from cubist pictures and the drawings produced by my daughters when they were toddlers. Furthermore, I take it that the ambitions of analyses of depiction are open-ended: they are meant to identify conditions that are, in each possible world, necessary and sufficient for being a picture that depicts a so-and-so.

Analyses of depiction therefore face a significant challenge. A correct analysis of depiction 'must explain the full range of [actual and possible] pictorial styles and types'.[8] Someone might, for example, formulate an analysis of depiction that identifies some conditions that are necessary and sufficient for something to be a picture which depicts a so-and-so in the general way that paintings from the High Renaissance tended to depict things. But the analysis is incorrect if one of the conditions is not necessary for something to be a picture that depicts a so-and-so in the general way that the drawings produced by my daughters when they were toddlers tended to depict things. Analyses of depiction are thus subject to a testing 'diversity constraint'.[9]

Semantic heterogeneity

The class of representational pictures in general is obviously very variegated. How profound are the variations in its members? In particular, do different types of representational pictures ever have contents of importantly different sorts?

A recurrent theme in detailed developmental studies of children's drawings is that, in the normal run of things, children move from producing pictures which are not meant to capture how things look to ones that

---

familiar concepts, rather than familiar concepts themselves: he argues that 'audio recordings are pictorial representations of the audible properties of things' (2006, 109–10), for instance.

[8] Lopes 1996, 32.
[9] Lopes 1996, 32.

are meant to do that. So, Luquet famously distinguished a stage at which children's drawings are guided by 'intellectual realism'; a stage in which they seek to draw 'what they know', by trying to produce 'the most faithful and complete representation of the object'[10] in the light of their overall knowledge of the item's characteristics. That stage tends to be followed, he claimed, by a stage whose guiding principle is 'visual realism'; a stage in which children attempt to draw 'what they see', by trying to capture how things look from a point of view.

Numerous other writers have made similar suggestions.[11] The general theme that the proposals share is likely to appeal to anyone who has spent time observing young children enthusiastically drawing pictures like Figure 6.1. For any attempt to treat that drawing as showing things as looking certain ways will be very strained.

The picture was certainly meant to record some parts of a rabbit using correlative marks. The reference to an eye is easy to spot, for example, and the sticking-out bit is meant to stand for a rabbit's ear; while the small curved line in the drawing's lower half stands for a mouth and the filled-in bit at the bottom stands for either a leg or the creature's tail. Yet it would be uncharitable to treat the picture as an attempt to represent the relevant bits of a rabbit by showing what they look like. It is rather an arrangement of pictorial symbols that just stand for undetached rabbit-parts, in the way that the symbols on a diagram or a map may just stand for things, where the spatial arrangement of the symbols also reflects some aspects of the spatial arrangement of a rabbit's body.

---

[10] Luquet [1927] 2001, 122.

[11] See Chapter 13 of Willats 1997 for a survey of some of the literature concerning the development of children's drawings. Willats's own view is that the earliest children's drawings 'use a system in which [marked] regions [of the surface upon which the child is drawing] stand for whole volumes', where 'the fundamental shape property represented . . . is extendedness, and topological properties like touching and enclosure are used to represent the spatial relations between parts of objects' (1997, 310). Crucially, according to Willats 1997, 318, the drawings which children produce at this earliest stage are (to use some phrases which Willats borrows from Marr) derived from 'object-centred' rather than 'viewer-centred' descriptions of the represented items; that is, from viewpoint-independent characterizations of the objects. But, as children get older, so they typically start using marked regions of the drawn-upon surface to represent 'edges and contours', where the resulting representations are in addition derived from viewer-centred descriptions of the represented things. Again, then, we have an account according to which the drawings generally produced by young children do not attempt to show us how things look.

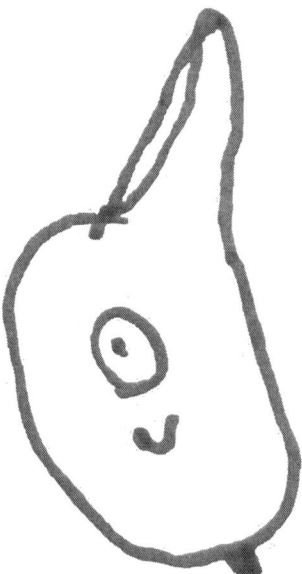

Figure 6.1. A rabbit, by a toddler

The representation of a mouth is based on a pictorial symbol that the artist had developed for the representation of human mouths, for instance. But the drawing does not represent a rabbit as having a mouth that looks human. Similarly, the representation of an eye uses a pictorial symbol that was once the artist's standard way of effecting pictorial references to eyes, whether in humans or animals. But she was not under the misapprehension that the eyes of all creatures look the same. Nor did she think that a rabbit's mouth is closer to its rear than to its ear.

Another example: Picasso spent the summer of 1910 in Cadaqués in Spain, producing pictures of typical cubist subjects like mandolins, guitarists, and women.[12] The experience of viewing the resulting pictures is redolent of the experience of viewing pictures which show how things look, for sure. It is hard not to slip into treating one's views of the pictures as disclosing things as looking certain ways involving variously angled planes, across which there are patterns of light and shade. And one can sometimes interpret parts of the pictures as signifying familiar things,

---

[12] See Palau i Fabre 1990, 179–95, for reproductions of many of the relevant pictures.

particularly when helped along by an awareness of the pictures' pictorial antecedents.

But the pictures are, in the end, stubbornly resistant to construal as distinctively visual representations. When one takes in its entirety the substantial oil painting of a guitarist that Picasso produced in Cadaqués, say, it just does not add up to a representation which shows things as looking certain ways.[13] One's experience of viewing the image thus forefronts some of the processes of interpretation which we tend to apply to pictures that themselves look certain ways, yet which do not make good sense of the painting itself.[14]

One response to the cases just discussed, and to the very many additional instances which could have been provided,[15] would be to claim that the pictures 'represent' but do not genuinely *depict* things. But the notion of depiction has no more to it than the idea that a picture depicts whatever it represents in a characteristically pictorial way.[16] And Figure 6.1, say, certainly represents a rabbit at the most fundamental and straightforwardly pictorial level, given the type of picture that it is: the picture consists of an assemblage of marks whose sole purpose is to stand for a rabbit and various

[13]   See Palau i Fabre 1990, 193, for the picture cited in the text.

[14]   According to the very influential 'semiotic' approach to cubism associated with Bois and Krauss, 'the turning point for Cubism' (Foster et al. 2004, 112) occurred in 1912, when Picasso began producing collages. At this moment, Picasso's creations supposedly start to reflect his realization of various general semiological theses; he shows, for example, a 'full comprehension of the consequences of [the arbitrariness of signs], namely, the differential nature of the sign and its mode of exchangeability based on its value' (Bois 1992, 175; see also Krauss 1992, the entry for 1912 in Foster et al. 2004, and, for some critical discussion, Chapter 4 of Karmel 2003). Whatever the virtues of this approach to cubism, its thoroughly semiotic nature—in particular, its exclusive concentration on how signs signify as opposed to the nature of their contents—means that it bypasses various issues relating exclusively to the latter. The approach consequently overlooks, for example, the possibility that the changes in 1912 are interestingly linked to a prior shift in the nature of the contents possessed by the pictures that Picasso and Braque had been producing.

[15]   Bahn's 1998 survey of prehistoric art is stuffed with pictures that do not seem to be amenable to treatment as distinctively visual representations, for example. Another interesting range of cases are the pictures which blind people sometimes produce using their senses of touch; see, for instance, Lopes 1997 and Hopkins 2000 for further discussion.

[16]   Abell says, for instance, that '[d]epiction is the form of representation that distinguishes figurative from abstract paintings' (2009, 183). And Hopkins asks 'What is pictorial representation? What is the form of representation which pictures display, and how does it differ from representation in language? Much of this book [Hopkins 1998] will be spent trying to understand this form of representation, which I shall for variety's sake consider under several names—"pictorial representation", "depiction" and "picturing"' (1998, 7–9). Neither of those entirely typical formulations bars Figure 6.1, say, from depicting a rabbit.

parts thereof. Related points apply to the Picasso painting cited previously and to very many further examples.

It thus seems clear that there are depictive pictures that are not distinctively visual representations. That is fine, as far as I am concerned. For I do not aim to base an analysis of depiction upon the theory of distinctively sensory content developed earlier. But the semantic variations found among depictive pictures are of more potential relevance to those who do hope to analyse depiction, for reasons that are explored in the following section.[17]

Analyses of distinctively visual picturing

Recent philosophical work on pictures has been dominated by the notion of depiction. More specifically, a lot of it has aimed to identify a correct analysis of depiction. The notion of depiction is meant to capture a characteristically pictorial version of the idea of aboutness. Yet our philosophical understanding of, say, language would have been greatly reduced if philosophers studying language had largely concentrated their efforts on developing 'analyses of linguistic aboutness'. One might wonder, by analogy, whether the concept of depiction provides a helpful focus for philosophical investigations into pictures.

Putative facts about what linguistic representations are 'about' often provide a helpful starting point for thinking about language. If one is to get a better grip on philosophical issues concerning linguistic representation, however, one needs quickly to leave the notion of aboutness behind. One needs to develop theoretical machinery—like, say, Frege's distinction between sense and reference, or the distinction between denoting expressions and predicates—which enables us to replace our relatively crude and messy assessments of what bits of language are about with more refined claims concerning their significance.

Once one has done all that, though, the notion of linguistic aboutness looks like a primitive precursor of the resulting ideas. And the really important task then seems to be to understand what it is for linguistic

---

[17] While I think that there are clearly pictures that are not distinctively visual representations, others may disagree. But whoever is right about that, I should emphasize that the main point of the following section still stands: we may make philosophical progress in studying pictures by, first, replacing mere talk of what pictures depict with more refined accounts of the natures of the contents that pictures may possess and then, second, basing our examinations of pictures on the resulting ideas.

expressions to have the various more refined forms of significance that
have superseded the idea of linguistic aboutness. Attempts to understand
what it is for a proper name to refer to some item proliferate, for instance;
but analyses of linguistic aboutness per se are thin on the ground. Aren't
parallel considerations likely to apply to pictures and depiction?[18]

The above worries are not just programmatic. The Watteau drawing
reproduced in Chapter 4 as Figure 4.5 depicts a man of a certain kind
because, in showing things as looking certain ways, the picture thereby
shows a man of the relevant type. More precisely, the picture depicts a
man because its distinctively visual content incorporates a way for things to
look whose appearance-content involves a certain sort of man, in accordance with the principle that *scene-showing corresponds to seeing*. By contrast,
the sorts of reasons on account of which the child's drawing of a rabbit
reproduced as Figure 6.1 depicts a rabbit are not the same, as the drawing
does not have a distinctively visual content.

More generally, facts about what pictures depict sometimes derive from
facts about the distinctively visual contents that the pictures possess. But
some depictive pictures do not have distinctively visual contents. In those
last cases, facts about what the pictures depict evidently do not derive from
facts about the distinctively visual contents that the pictures possess. The
semantic heterogeneity in the class of depictive pictures therefore generates a corresponding heterogeneity in the representational facts that provide the bases for truths about what different sorts of pictures depict.

To capture the kinds of variations just described, one must start investigating pictures in the light of the different sorts of contents that they may
possess.[19] But that project requires one to shift one's attention away from
the class of depictive pictures as a whole. Perhaps we will eventually be

---

[18] Hyman argues that philosophical work on pictures has often suffered greatly from a
failure to attend to pictorial analogues of Frege's distinction between sense and reference
(Hyman forthcoming). More generally, and in agreement with some of the themes in the
current section, Hyman notes that philosophers studying pictorial representation have been
prone to work with rather crude semantic tools, particularly compared to philosophers
studying linguistic representations.

[19] Lopes seems to acknowledge this sort of point; he 'enumerates four varieties of depiction', saying that 'there are four ways in which pictures can refer, there are four varieties of
pictorial sense, and understanding a picture as the kind of picture it is means tracing its
reference to its subject in the appropriate way' (Lopes 1996, 172). I am, though, doubtful of
Lopes's further claim that '[r]ecognition is involved in all pictorial representation; it is what
distinguishes the meaning of pictures from that of other kinds of representation' (1996, 173);
see below for further discussion. (The second part of the statement just quoted seems also to

able to construct an overarching analysis of depiction in general, by amalgamating correct accounts of what it is to be a picture that possesses one sort of content rather than another. But perhaps not; maybe, for instance, the class of depictive pictures is just too messy for that. That would hardly matter, though, if we have anyway come to a clear understanding of the more basic representational facts about pictures that we track using our assessments of what they depict.

The range of pictures that possess distinctively visual contents forms one very significant portion of the class of depictive pictures as a whole. The distinction between the depictive pictures that have distinctively visual contents and the depictive pictures that do not have distinctively visual contents is important enough that it ought to be captured by any comprehensive philosophical account of pictorial representation. Whatever happens to the project of analysing depiction in general, then, here is another worthwhile enterprise: to explain what it is for something to be a picture that shows things as looking a certain way.

One who seeks to explain what it is for something to be a picture that shows things as looking a certain way attempts to provide a *correct analysis of distinctively visual picturing*. A correct analysis of distinctively visual picturing would tell us exactly when an item counts as a picture that shows things as looking a certain way. More precisely, it would identify, for each way that a picture may show things as looking, some conditions that are necessary and sufficient for an item's being a picture that shows things as looking that way.[20]

Analytical alternatives

Imagine that someone has developed an incorrect analysis of depiction. Yet suppose that the analysis is not hopeless. Suppose, more specifically,

conflate putative special features of the ways in which we *grasp* the contents of pictures with putative special features of those contents themselves.)

[20] As defined in the text, correct analyses of distinctively visual picturing may leave important questions unanswered. So, suppose that a certain picture shows things as looking way *T*. A correct analysis of distinctively visual picturing might identify some conditions whose satisfaction by the picture are necessary and sufficient for its showing things as looking way *T*, without settling whether the picture shows things as looking way *T* from a perspective or in the course of a visual sensation. Correct analyses of distinctively visual picturing may thus beg to be further refined, to capture additional crucial facts about the contents of distinctively visual pictures. Analyses of distinctively visual picturing will nonetheless serve as a useful focus for subsequent discussion.

that the analysis seems to work well for certain pictures but that it hits problems when faced by some other pictures that seem to be rather different from the first lot. While the person has not produced a correct analysis of depiction in general, the analysis might still be very useful. For maybe it can tell us important things about what it is to be a picture that possesses one important kind of content. In particular, it would be worth considering whether the analysis might lead us to a correct analysis of distinctively visual picturing.

Analyses of depiction do seem often to be driven by a primary concern with *distinctively visual pictures*—by a primary concern with pictures that show things as looking certain ways. And that is hardly surprising, as distinctively visual pictures are particularly prevalent within our culture.

Abell's analysis of depiction, for instance, includes a condition that captures the general thought that '[t]o depict an object, a marked surface must resemble it in respects that jointly capture its overall appearance';[21] while Hopkins identifies various supposed features of picturing in general that are 'captured, loosely but suggestively, in the thought that depictions represent things through representing their [visual] appearances'.[22] The thoughts driving Abell's condition and Hopkins's comment seem to fit well with many obvious examples of distinctively visual pictures; they sit easily with all of the images reproduced in Chapter 4, for instance. But there any many other kinds of pictures in relation to which they are far less clearly correct. Similar remarks apply to a range of further ideas that philosophers have deployed in seeking to analyse depiction in general, as we will see below.

When a philosopher develops an analysis of depiction, certain pictures commonly appear to sit uneasily with the general conception of pictorial representation that prompted the analysis. The pictures are consequently treated as peripheral cases. Now that we have isolated the class of distinctively visual pictures, though, another way of responding to such challenging examples may sometimes be available: one might scale back one's analytical ambitions somewhat, by reformulating one's analysis of depiction as an analysis of distinctively visual picturing. As later sections of this chapter will make clear, I think that some well-known philosophical approaches to depiction in general would benefit from being transformed in that manner.

---

[21] Abell 2009, 218.   [22] Hopkins 1998, 48.

Metaphysically ambitious analyses

Reconsider the following passage, which was quoted above: '[p]hiloso-phical accounts of depiction aim, first and foremost, to answer the meta-physical question of what it is for one thing to depict another. That is, they aim to provide individually necessary and jointly sufficient conditions for being a picture of some object.'[23]

Answers to the metaphysical question of what it is to be a picture of some object need to earn our respect, by illuminating suitable matters of philosophical interest. The successful identification of some conditions that obtain just in case an item is a picture of something is not in itself particularly worthwhile. Philosophers have thus sometimes attempted to substantiate their analyses of depiction by appealing to the theoretical work that they can do. In particular, they have sometimes appealed to *explanations*.

The philosophical gains which may result from paying attention to the explanatory powers of analyses of depiction are stressed most forcefully by Hopkins.[24] Hopkins argues that his analysis of depiction smoothly explains a host of general facts about depiction,[25] such as the facts that '[e]verything depicted is depicted from some point of view',[26] that '[w]hatever can be depicted can [apparently] be seen',[27] and that '[t]here is . . . no *bare* depic-tion of particulars'.[28] Budd also aims to use his own related analysis of depiction to explain why 'depiction must always be from a point of

---

[23] Abell and Bantinaki 2010, 2. Abell also distinguishes 'the epistemological question of how we are able to work out that one thing depicts another' (2009, 184).

[24] Hopkins emphasizes explanatory matters on, for example, pp. 23–4 of Hopkins 1998; see also Hopkins 1995. Budd also points out that '[a] theory of depiction derives its support from its ability to explain salient facts about pictures and to make sense of pre-theoretical intuitions' (Budd 1993, 392).

[25] My own view is that the various supposed general features of depiction cited shortly are not in fact general features of depiction; they are merely general features of distinctively visual picturing. So, for instance, the thought that depiction must always be perspectival makes good sense if one holds that depictive pictures 'represent things through representing their [visual] appearances'. For visual appearances are always perspectival. Yet some depictive pictures are not distinctively visual pictures. And it is hard to see why one would hold that those last pictures must depict whatever they depict in a perspectival manner. (From where does Figure 6.1 depict the rabbit that it depicts, for instance? It seems to me that there is nothing perspectival in the way that Figure 6.1 stands for a rabbit, just as there is often nothing perspectival in the way that the symbols on diagrams and maps stand for things.)

[26] Hopkins 1998, 27.

[27] Hopkins 1998, 28; see Chapter 1 for discussion of the inserted 'apparently'.

[28] Hopkins 1998, 24.

view';[29] while Abell seeks to use her 'intention-based resemblance' analysis of depiction to explain the supposed features of depiction in general
upon which Hopkins concentrates.[30]

Suppose that an analysis of distinctively visual picturing is meant to
answer the metaphysical question what it is to be a picture that shows
things as looking a certain way. Then the analysis is *metaphysically ambitious*.
We might reasonably hope that metaphysically ambitious analyses of
distinctively visual picturing will generate explanations of various facts.
But just what sorts of explanations should we expect them to provide?

Care needs to be taken in answering that question. In particular,
philosophical theorizing about types of representations should be informed
by an awareness of the distinction between the following two sets of
phenomena. First, there are those phenomena that can be explained just
in terms of the nature of the contents which the relevant representations
possess. Second, there are those phenomena whose explanations need
more than theories of content for the representations can provide.

Some of the most striking general features of distinctively visual picturing simply reflect the distinctively sensory nature of the contents belonging
to distinctively visual pictures. We saw in Chapter 3, for instance, that the
perspectival manner in which distinctively visual pictures show things to us
merely reflects the distinctively visual nature of their contents, along with
the principle that *scene-showing corresponds to seeing*. The same applies to
the fact that distinctively visual pictures can only show items that may look
to be present as having properties that may look to be instantiated. Indeed,
we saw in Chapter 3 that an open-ended array of further general facts
about distinctively visual pictures may be explained just by citing the
distinctively sensory nature of their contents.

Some central features of distinctively visual picturing may thus be accommodated without the use of analyses of distinctively visual picturing, for they
may be satisfactorily explained using this book's theory of distinctively
sensory content alone.[31] There are many other explanatory jobs available

[29] Budd 1993, 392.

[30] Abell 2009, 218–21. See Abell 2009, 217, for the full version of her analysis.

[31] Gregory 2010b explores this point at more length, although the various features of
distinctively visual picturing considered in that paper are there wrongly identified with
features of depiction in general. (That paper also ignores the distinction between sensation-
characterizing and perspective-characterizing distinctively sensory contents, concentrating
entirely upon the latter.)

for metaphysically ambitious analyses of distinctively visual picturing, however. The next section identifies one major task for them to perform.

Bridging the divide between appearance and content

Metaphysically ambitious analyses of distinctively visual picturing aim to elucidate individual circumstances using general conditions. They should tell us why *this* particular thing—having as it does *these* properties—counts as a picture that shows things as looking certain specific ways. But one who appreciates that a picture shows things as looking certain ways is surely responding at some level to the properties on account of which the picture does show things as looking those ways. The properties in virtue of which distinctively visual pictures show things as looking various ways must therefore somehow be linked to the visible characteristics of the pictures which lead us to grasp the ways that they show things as looking.

That last observation can be used to generate a useful and relatively refined way of comparing metaphysically ambitious analyses of distinctively visual picturing. Suppose that some metaphysically ambitious analysis of distinctively visual picturing states that an item is a distinctively visual picture that shows things as looking way *T* just in case the item satisfies the set of conditions *C*. And suppose that another metaphysically ambitious analysis of distinctively visual picturing states that an item is a distinctively visual picture that shows things as looking way *T* just in case the thing satisfies the different set of conditions *C**.

Imagine next that we appreciate that a distinctively visual picture shows things as looking way *T*, on the basis of the fact that the picture itself looks certain ways to us. *Distinctively sensory showing comes from subjective informativeness.* Hence, our awareness that the picture shows things as looking way *T* involves a subjectively informative identification of *T* on the basis of the way that the picture itself looks to us: it involves a vision-based identification of *T* in terms of what it is like to have *T*-sensations.

According to one analysis, the picture shows things as looking way *T* on account of the picture's satisfaction of the conditions *C*. Yet according to the other analysis, the critical conditions are *C**. Suppose that we are best able to explain how the picture's satisfaction of *C* is relevant to our vision-based subjectively informative identification of *T*. Then, other things being equal, we should favour the metaphysically ambitious analysis that appeals to C over the one that appeals to C^*. For the former analysis enables us better to understand how the properties which form the basis for the picture's distinctively visual significance are connected to our understanding of the thing.

The above paragraph does not provide us with a full set of resources with which to assess metaphysically ambitious analyses of distinctively visual picturing. For there are other equally significant dimensions of assessment: metaphysically ambitious analyses need to be correct, for one thing. But any account of what it is to be a picture that shows things as looking some way should play its part in an explanation of how we manage to identify the ways that distinctively visual pictures show things as looking on the basis of the ways that the pictures themselves look to us; or, as I shall put it, in an explanation of how we *bridge the divide between appearance and content*.

The remaining three sections of this chapter use that point to compare some possible approaches to the analysis of distinctively visual picturing.[32] Each of the approaches to be considered is a counterpart of a well-known approach to the analysis of depiction in general.[33]

Recognition

Our dealings with pictures often call upon our ability to recognize things by sight. You may recognize your parents in a photo, for example; or you

---

[32] A further clarification: suppose a person views some item, rightly taking the thing to be a picture that shows things as looking way T. Here is one question: why is the person led to identify T in terms of what it is like to have T-sensations, upon viewing the item? And here is another question: how is the person able to know, upon viewing the item and consequently identifying T in terms of what it is like to have T-sensations, that the item is actually a picture that shows things as looking way T? (Why doesn't the person simply take herself to have responded to the item in an idiosyncratic fashion, for instance?) The first of those questions, rather than the second, is the chief focus of the following sections.

[33] Note that the range of approaches explored below is not meant to be comprehensive. In particular, I have not discussed whether there might be some way of adapting the kind of positions on depiction developed in Goodman 1969 and Kulvicki 2006 to generate a metaphysically ambitious analysis of distinctively visual picturing that will help us understand how our views of pictures enable us to make subjectively informative identifications of ways that the pictures show things as looking. Nor have I discussed the prospects for attempts to analyse distinctively visual picturing using mere objective resemblances between pictures and their subjects rather than experienced resemblances (Hyman 2006 favours objective resemblances over experienced ones, for instance).

may realize that a picture displays a curlew because you have learned to recognize curlews in the past. Some philosophers have sought to base theoretical accounts of depiction upon visual recognitional capacities, by appealing to the parts played by the latter in enabling people to interpret pictures correctly.

It is clear that our ability to interpret pictures correctly is often informed by the sorts of pictures that we have actually encountered. The kinds of items that are depicted in cubist still life paintings may be wholly obscure to someone who has never viewed cubist pictures before, for instance. But with a little training the person may become quite adept at spotting references to, say, wine glasses and violins within the pictures. More generally, it is often natural to treat pictures as belonging to groups whose members depict what they depict in broadly the same sort of way, and to treat our ability to understand particular pictures as involving familiarities with the workings of relevant groups of pictures.

All this has suggested to some philosophers that individual pictures should generally be viewed as belonging to broader pictorial systems. Now, there are various ways in which one might attempt to divide pictures up into systems. Schier emphasizes the relationships which our abilities to understand pictures may bear to one another, for instance;[34] but Lopes appeals to general semantic properties that pictures may share.[35] Both Schier and Lopes nonetheless share a certain overall view of the way in which depiction fundamentally works. For they both claim that visual recognitional capacities are fundamental to facts about what is depicted by the specific pictures that belong to pictorial systems.

Suppose that someone has acquired the ability to grasp the contents of pictures in, say, the pictorial system to which Mannerist paintings generally belong. Imagine that the person encounters Parmigianino's *Madonna of the Long Neck* for the first time. Then the person should be able to tell pretty quickly that the picture depicts a woman, just because the viewer can presumably reliably recognize women by sight. Likewise, the person will probably be able to spot that the picture depicts a pillar, as the person is probably able visually to recognize pillars. More generally, Schier and Lopes make the following claim: the range of items that are depicted by Parmigianino's painting maps onto the range of visual recognitional

---

[34] Schier 1986, 47–8. [35] Lopes 1996, 127–31.

capacities with which the picture may engage, when it is viewed by people who are familiar with the pictorial system to which it belongs.

So, Schier states that '[i]f S depicts O that is because an ability to recognise O could be enough, given an initiation into the relevant symbol system, to explain differentially P's getting his interpretation of S right'.[36] And Lopes says, 'in sum, that pictures embody information enabling viewers to recognize their contents and their subjects. The recognition skills we bring to pictures depend on and extend the dynamic recognition skills exercised in ordinary perception'.[37] (He claims, too, that '[p]ictorial competence is system-relative'.[38]) Schier builds an analysis of depiction in general upon the foregoing ideas,[39] while Lopes aims to use them to identify an especially primitive mode of pictorial representation that he calls 'basic depiction'.[40]

Do visual recognitional capacities have much potential as the cornerstones of a metaphysically ambitious analysis of distinctively visual picturing? Look around you. Given the way that things now look to you, your knowledge of what things look like means that you are able to classify lots of what you can see. You may recognize that you are surrounded by fine furniture, for instance; perhaps you recognize your trusty *chaise longue*. But your visual recognitional capacities are there responding to the way that things look to you: the way that things look to you is not itself somehow merely constituted by the workings of your visual recognitional capacities.[41]

Related points apply to distinctively visual pictures. Review one of the images in Chapter 4. Your appreciation of the ways that the picture shows things as looking, along with your knowledge of what things look like, means that you recognize that the picture shows items of various sorts. Again, however, your visual recognitional capacities are there responding to something else: to your subjectively informative identifications of ways that the picture shows things as looking, on the basis of the ways that the picture itself looks to you. Yet what we currently seek to understand just is how those last identifications are effected. And simply appealing to your knowledge of what things look like is not going to help us to do that.

---

[36] Schier 1986, 49.   [37] Lopes 1996, 149.
[38] Lopes 1996, 149.   [39] Schier 1986, 115–16.   [40] Lopes 1996, 151–6.
[41] That is not to deny that your visual recognitional capacities may somehow affect the ways that things may look to you, of course.

More generally, suppose that one concentrates upon the *language* which we ordinarily use to make claims about what distinctively visual pictures depict. Then our visual recognitional capacities might well seem somehow to form the basis of picturing. After all, our knowledge of what things look like evidently does often guide our talk about what is depicted by pictures that show things as looking certain ways. My realization that some photo 'shows a tackhead banjo' depends upon my ability to recognize tackhead banjos by sight, for instance.

Once one acknowledges that facts about what distinctively visual pictures depict are determined by facts concerning the ways that the pictures show things as looking, though, our capacities for visual recognition recede into the background. The capacities are important, of course: they allow us to classify conceptually the items that are shown in the pictures, on the basis of our appreciations of the ways that the pictures show things as looking. But the recognition-based classifications which we thereby accomplish thus rest upon more primitive modes of interaction with pictures.[42] In particular, they rest upon our prior ability to identify types of visual sensations in subjectively informative ways, on the basis of the ways that pictures themselves look to us. That is, they rest upon our prior ability to bridge the divide between appearance and content.

It therefore seems that a major explanatory shortcoming will afflict any attempt to model a metaphysically ambitious analysis of distinctively visual picturing upon the approaches to depiction developed by Schier and Lopes: the analysis would be forced to rely upon mental operations that work with, but do not themselves implement, subjectively informative identifications of ways for things to look; and so the analysis would be unable to provide a satisfying explanation of how we manage to bridge the divide between appearance and content. Other theoretical accounts of depiction in general are based upon mental processes that can themselves yield subjectively informative identifications of ways for things to look, however; the next section considers one such case.

---

[42] A relative of the point made in the text seems in fact to be implicit in some of Lopes's remarks. He says, for example, that '[a] picture is a representation *that embodies information on the basis of which* its source can be identified by a suitably equipped perceiver' (1996, 151; emphasis added).

Pretence

Pictures often enrich our imaginative lives. There must be few attentive visitors to art galleries who have not found themselves drawn into day-dreams by the images on display. But are our imaginative capacities central to our ability to comprehend pictures? The current section briefly explores the explanatory potential of an analysis of distinctively visual picturing that is based upon Walton's approach to depiction in general, an approach that accords a special place to our imaginations.

Walton's account of depiction is embedded within an attempt to use the idea of 'make-believe' to elucidate an impressively wide array of phenomena. He claims that many familiar activities may be better understood by appreciating the part that pretence plays in them. In particular, Walton holds that we are all party to a game—let's call it the *picture-game*—in which the things that we call 'pictures' play a crucial role. And he holds that the fact that something plays the relevant role in the game is what makes it a depictive picture.

The picture-game involves our looking at pictures and then imagining the very visual sensations which we thereby enjoy to be visual sensations in which we are seeing what the pictures depict. Walton claims, for instance, that '[a] picture of a turtle is a prop in games in which viewers imagine seeing a turtle, and imagine their actual visual experience of the picture to be their seeing of a turtle. It is fictional, in the world of the game, that a turtle is an object of their vision'.[43]

Walton presents his theory as an analysis of depiction.[44] But it is worth considering whether it converts into a decent metaphysically ambitious analysis of distinctively visual picturing, partly because the theory seems somewhat unpromising when it is applied to many of the depictive pictures that do not show things as looking certain ways. When I view the toddler's drawing of a rabbit reproduced as Figure 6.1, for example, I find myself bamboozled by the demand to pretend that the very visual sensations that the picture affords me are views of a rabbit.[45]

Here is a Waltonian analysis of distinctively visual picturing:

---

[43] Walton 2008, 74.   [44] Walton 1990, 296.

[45] Walton writes that 'pictures capture the *appearance* of the things they picture' (2008, 65) at one point, so it may be that Walton's thought about pictures has been guided by a focus upon distinctively visual pictures. (The context of the remark just quoted suggests that it may be coming from an imaginary interlocutor; but Walton does not take issue with it.)

(6.A)   An item is a picture that shows things as looking way T just in case viewers who are playing the picture-game are to imagine their views of the item as being visual sensations of type T.

To what extent does (6.A) help us to understand how we pass from our views of distinctively visual pictures to our subjectively informative identifications of the ways that the pictures show things as looking?

There are lots of ways in which imaginings may identify ways for things to look. I have no idea what my brother and sister are doing at this moment, but I may nonetheless imagine the way that things currently look to my brother to be exactly the way that things currently look to my sister. That imagining did not identify a way for things to look in terms of what it is like for things to look that way; that is, the imagining's content did not single out a way for things to look in a subjectively informative manner. An account of our ability to bridge the divide between appearance and content will therefore need to move beyond our wholly general ability to imagine things as looking certain ways.

More specifically, suppose that (6.A) is to help us understand how we bridge the divide between appearance and content. Then the contents of the imaginings cited in the principle need to be restricted somewhat. The imaginings must be ones in which, first, we imagine visual sensations to be ones in which things look certain ways; where, second, the imaginings single out the relevant ways for things to look in terms of what it is like to have visual sensations in which things look those ways. How useful is (6.A) once that restriction is imposed?

Bearing in mind the points made in the previous two paragraphs, the imaginative processes cited by (6.A) may look like a promising basis for explaining how we are able to bridge the divide between appearance and content. Produce a visual mental image, for instance: let's say that your visual mental image shows things as looking like *that*. Suppose that some picture also shows things as looking like *that*. Assume that someone views the picture and imagines the visual sensations that she is enjoying to be ones in which things look like *that*. Then the person has apparently passed from her view of the picture to a subjectively informative identification of a way that the picture shows things as looking.

Yet why did the previous person's imagining relate to that particular way for things to look, rather than to some other one? The answer to the previous question will presumably advert to the manner in which the precise content of the person's imagining was shaped by the way that the picture looked to her as she viewed it. But the question is therefore itself one of the main questions that we need to answer if we are to get a clear view of how our person bridged the divide between appearance and content.

One might try to explain within a Waltonian framework why the person's imagining related to a particular way for things to look, by appealing to the person's appreciation of the rules of the picture-game. It might be said that the picture-game involves rules that connect, first, the ways that appropriate pictures themselves look to, second, subjectively informative identifications of correlative ways for things to look. The person then applies those rules to the ways that the relevant picture looks to her as she sees it. And her application of the rules leads her to imagine that the visual sensations she is having are ones in which things look the correlated ways, where the person's use of the rules leads her to identify those last ways for things to look using subjectively informative modes of presentation.

But that response hardly amounts to progress. In particular, we need now to understand the nature of the relevant rules and how our person 'applies' them to yield her awareness of ways that the picture shows things as looking. How exactly do the rules map ways that pictures look onto subjectively informative identifications of corresponding ways for things to look? And what sorts of mental processes are involved in the person's 'applying' the rules to produce subjectively informative versions of the rather peculiar imaginings cited by (6.A)?[46]

Whether or not the Waltonian analysis of distinctively visual picturing embodied in (6.A) is correct,[47] it thus does very little to help us understand

---

[46] Walton insists that the 'visual games of make-believe' which underpin our understandings of pictures 'must be sufficiently *rich* and *vivid* visually', where '[t]hey are rich to the extent that they allow for the fictional performance of a large variety of visual actions, by virtue of actually performing visual actions vis à vis the work' and '[a] game's (visual) *vivacity* consists in the vivacity with which the participant imagines performance of the visual actions which fictionally he performs' (1990, 296). The restriction to 'rich and vivid' games does not address the issues raised in the text, however: the talk of 'richness' just raises the question what determines the nature of the large variety of visual actions that we are to imagine ourselves performing when we view pictures; while the talk of 'vivacity' sounds like a gesture at the fact that our comprehending views of distinctively visual pictures involve an awareness of what it is like to have visual sensations in which things look the ways that the pictures show things as looking.

[47] For what it is worth, I think that the analysis is incorrect: the claim that our appreciations of the ways that pictures show things as looking occur against the backdrop of a 'picture-game' that prescribes the sorts of recondite imaginings specified in (6.A) just seems to me quite

how we bridge the divide between appearance and content. The analysis perhaps improves upon the recognitional approach examined in the previous section, by invoking mental processes that may themselves yield subjectively informative identifications of ways for things to look. But the analysis leaves us in the dark as to how the ways that distinctively visual pictures look to us shape the particular subjectively informative identifications that are involved in our understandings of the pictures.

Experienced resemblances

It has seemed to many people that there is something phenomenologically distinctive about those episodes in which we see pictures 'as pictures', although it is a special subjective character which the episodes share with some of our visual encounters with other things. When viewing a jumble of shadows, for example, we can sometimes discern beings like dragons in the accidental shapes assumed by the shadows. And such experiences of seeing items in shadows have a felt flavour that is also present when, say, we suddenly come to see some painted marks on a canvas as forming a picture of a person.

Wollheim is the philosopher most responsible for the part that 'seeing-in' experiences have played within current philosophical debates about picturing. He claims that seeing-in experiences are 'twofolded', in that during them one is 'visually aware of the surface [one looks] at, and [one] discerns something standing out in front of, or (in certain cases) receding behind, something else'. He states, too, that the two folds of seeing-in experiences are 'distinguishable but also inseparable',[48] and that the two-foldedness of seeing-in experiences makes their special phenomenology 'incommensurate'[49] with that of more ordinary visual sensations.

Wollheim's insistence on the *sui generis* nature of seeing-in makes his approach a rather unpromising source of explanations of how the ways that pictures look to us generate our subjectively informative identifications of ways that the pictures show things as looking. But other writers have been more hopeful about the possibility of anatomizing seeing-in. In

far-fetched. (I think that Walton's analysis of depiction in general is incorrect, for the same pretty crude reason.)

[48] This quotation and the previous one are from Wollheim 1987, 46.
[49] Wollheim 1987, 47.

particular, some philosophers have identified seeing-in experiences with episodes in which we experience ways that things look to us as being similar to other ways for things to look.

Budd and Hopkins have developed approaches of this kind, as has Peacocke.[50] I shall concentrate upon Budd's ideas in what follows, although the points to be made below could have been illustrated using either Hopkins's or Peacocke's views instead. Budd builds his analysis of depiction upon the concept of the *visual field* that forms part of a particular visual sensation: 'my visual field is just [the complete way the world is then represented to me by my visual experience] considered in abstraction from one of its three spatial dimensions, namely, distance outwards from my point of view'.[51]

To illustrate Budd's thinking here, suppose that you see a pair of railway tracks running straight off into the distance. Then your visual field—what results from subtracting any information relating to locations outwards from you from the total way that things look to you to be—does not characterize the tracks as being parallel. For the ascription of parallelism to the railway tracks, within the visual appearances that you are enjoying, rests upon the fact that those appearances situate the tracks as running directly *away* from you. In fact, as 'the angle subtended at [your] eyes by the width of the tracks gets less as they recede',[52] there is a sense in which your visual field presents the railway tracks as converging.

Now, if the ways that distinctively visual pictures themselves look are somehow often similar to the ways that they show things as looking, the crucial similarities will usually be fundamentally two-dimensional. Pictures generally look flat, even when the scenes that they are showing are not. But Budd's idea of a visual field is engineered to allow us to home in on precisely those aspects of the ways that things look to us which are purged of three-dimensionality. Hence one's views of a flat-looking picture may include a visual field that resembles the visual field that would form part of apparent views of the receding scene which the picture shows.

---

[50] See Peacocke 1987; Budd 1993; and Hopkins 1995 and 1998. Each of those writers connects their views to seeing-in: Budd writes that '[t]he crucial issue is the nature of the spectator's visual awareness of the picture-surface when he sees what a picture depicts' (1993, 158); Hopkins explicitly uses his approach to formulate a biconditional relating to seeing-in (1998, 77); and Peacocke says that his theory 'ought to be taken as an attempt to implement or meet the desiderata of those who have wanted to explain depiction by making reference to a particular kind of seeing' (1987, 401).

[51] Budd 1993, 158.   [52] Budd 1993, 159.

Suppose that, when viewing a picture, one's visual field resembles the visual field which would form part of one's visual experiences on some other occasion. That fact alone is not sufficient for seeing-in to take place. The experience of, say, seeing a person in a picture incorporates some kind of *awareness* of a relationship between what things are like for one in viewing the picture and what appropriate views of a person are like.

Budd therefore proposes that seeing-in experiences occur when, upon viewing a surface, one *experiences* one's visual field *as resembling* the visual field which would be incorporated in the views of some scene from a certain viewpoint.[53] As noted above, Hopkins and Peacocke also endorse 'experienced-resemblance' theories of seeing-in. Their accounts differ from Budd's with regard to the specific resemblances whose being experienced is supposedly responsible for seeing-in experiences. (Hopkins, for instance, argues that experienced resemblances in 'outline shape' form the 'distinctive core' of seeing-in.[54])

My own view is that Budd's approach—or indeed any other theory that takes seeing-in experiences as its starting point—cannot generate a correct analysis of depiction in general. For I think that there are many depictive pictures without distinctively visual contents that do not generate suitable seeing-in experiences in comprehending viewers. More generally, experienced-resemblance analyses of depiction seem to be prime examples of analyses of depiction in general that would benefit from being recast as analyses of distinctively visual picturing, for the following reasons.

I take it that experienced-resemblance approaches to depiction start from the following general idea: a picture depicts the sorts of items that feature in the ways for things to look that appropriately situated viewers of the picture experience their views of the picture itself as resembling.[55]

---

[53] See Budd 1993, 161. Budd's account in fact includes another condition, as he holds that seeing-in experiences 'must involve a visual awareness of the presence before you of a marked surface'. I think that Budd ought to drop this condition from his theory, but that fact is not responsible for its absence from the text (which is instead owed to its current irrelevance).

[54] For discussion of outline shape, see Hopkins 1998, 53–63. (Hopkins is happy to allow that other sorts of experienced resemblances are important to seeing-in, however (Hopkins 1998, 88).) Hyman employs the closely related concept of 'occlusion shape' in developing his own rather different approach to depiction (see Chapter 5 of Hyman 2006).

[55] The way that a certain distinctively visual picture looks might commonly be experienced as being similar to some other way for things to look, even though the latter way for things to look is not a way that the picture shows things as looking; in particular, the relevant

That starting point makes good sense when one just focuses upon distinctively visual pictures. For the contents of distinctively visual pictures do incorporate ways for things to look whose associated visual appearances determine what the pictures show. But many depictive pictures are not distinctively visual representations, and it is unclear why one would expect the previous ideas to apply to those pictures too.

No matter; it is easy to adapt Budd's analysis of depiction to generate an analysis of distinctively visual picturing:

> (6.B)   An item is a picture that shows things as looking way T just in case one who views the item in suitable circumstances will experience the visual field figuring in the resulting sensation as resembling the visual field that is common to visual sensations of type T.

What is added to (6.B) by the talk of 'experienced' resemblance?[56] Could the principle be rephrased without loss using, say, mere talk of resemblances that are 'known' to be present?

Imagine that, while watching some clouds drifting past, you experience your visual field as resembling the visual field that would figure in some apparent views of faces. Then you must surely be conscious of suitable similarities between, first, what things are now like visually for you and, second, what it is like apparently to see faces of certain sorts. For suppose that someone knows that the visual field figuring in the way that things look to her resembles the visual field that is common to the sensations of some kind, where the person nonetheless has no idea of what it is like to have sensations of the second variety. (Suppose that the person somehow knows that her current visual sensations are like those once enjoyed by a certain person, for instance, without knowing which aspects of the way that things look to her are responsible for the resemblances.) Then she has not actually *experienced* the first visual field as resembling the second.

---

resemblance might be entirely inadvertent. The statement made in the text therefore ought really to state that 'a picture depicts the sorts of items that feature in the ways for things to look that appropriately situated viewers of the picture experience—and are meant to experience—their views of the picture itself as resembling'. (Numerous writers have emphasized the need for the previous sort of qualification: see, for instance, Wollheim 1987, 47–8; and Budd 1993, 155–6.) I have ignored these issues in the text, for simplicity's sake.

[56] Section V of Budd 1993 examines some of the distinctively experiential aspects of his approach to seeing-in.

The experiences of resemblance cited in (6.B) thus incorporate subject-ively informative identifications of particular ways for things to look; and those identifications flow from the ways that things actually look to the relevant subjects. More generally, experienced-resemblance accounts of depiction rely upon our ability to be conscious of similarities between what things are actually like for us visually and what it is like to have visual sensations in which things look other ways. When that occurs, however, one's awareness of the relevant resemblances itself includes a subjectively informative identification of a way for things to look. And the resulting identification is based upon the apparently related way that things actually look to one.

Suppose, for instance, that you view a picture that shows things as looking way T while you are placed in suitable circumstances. Given (6.B), you will experience the visual field included in your view of the picture as resembling the visual field that is common to T-sensations. But the resulting experience of resemblance will itself incorporate an identification of T in terms of what it is like to have T-sensations. And that subjectively informative identification of T will be based upon the way that the picture itself looks to you. The assumed correctness of (6.B) therefore allows us very straightforwardly to account for your ability in that case to bridge the divide between appearance and content.[57]

Experienced-resemblance analyses of distinctively visual picturing thus promise to generate attractive explanations of how we manage to bridge the divide between appearance and content. And that is an important point in their favour, even if it is not sufficient to show that some experi-enced-resemblance analysis is best able to answer the metaphysical ques-tion what it is to be a picture which shows things as looking a certain way.[58] By contrast, the explanatory failings of the alternative analyses of distinctively visual picturing envisaged in the previous couple of sections

---

[57] Note that the ideas underlying (6.B) might be useful even if (6.B) is not a correct analysis of distinctively visual picturing. In particular, suppose that the conditions on the right-hand side of (6.B) are *sufficient* for an item's being a picture that shows things as looking way T. Then we might still be able to use a weaker relative of (6.B) to explain how we *sometimes* effect our vision-based subjectively informative identifications of ways that pictures show things as looking.

[58] I think that appropriate analyses of distinctively visual picturing in terms of objective resemblances between pictures and their subjects are probably able to replicate the explana-tory successes of experienced-resemblance analyses noted in the text, for instance.

count against their claims to be satisfying metaphysically ambitious analyses of distinctively visual picturing.

The foregoing discussions have illustrated some of the philosophically interesting matters that become visible when, putting aside the relatively undiscriminating concept of depiction, one treats distinctively visual picturing as a subject worthy of study in its own right. More generally, the former discussions combine with the previous chapter's conjectures concerning the neural bases of sensory mental imagery, to show how a pure theory of distinctively sensory content may play its part in helping us better to understand the ways in which distinctively sensory representations of various sorts express their distinctively sensory contents.

7

More on Pictures

Theoretical accounts of the contents belonging to pictures need to provide decent characterizations of the semantic features exhibited by pictures of different kinds. The current chapter shows how Chapter 3's theory of distinctively sensory content may be used to investigate some important varieties of distinctively visual pictures. The resulting discussions provide some further support for the theory, by further illustrating its utility. But the relatively undeveloped state of theorizing about pictorial content means that there is also just some intellectual interest in seeking better to understand the semantic complexities of distinctively visual pictures.

The bulk of the chapter develops a detailed account of an important aspect of the multifaceted idea of pictorial realism: the phenomenon of pictorial 'lifelikeness'. This phenomenon provides a particularly rich illustration of how the ways that pictures show things as looking may interact significantly with the ways that the pictures themselves look. The account of lifelikeness articulated below provides a refined articulation of the simple idea that the ways that lifelike pictures look to us are especially similar to the ways that they show things as looking. The account is compared to some alternative treatments of lifelikeness in the literature; it is also used to explain a host of important facts about lifelike pictures.

The chapter's final sections examine some of the interesting issues raised by the many pictures which are naturally construed as portraying visual episodes from the inside. Despite their relative obviousness, the questions examined do not appear previously to have been addressed in the literature. Their treatment illustrates how we may, while starting from anodyne observations about our understanding of pictures, use relatively detailed theorizing about distinctively visual content to lay bare surprising facets of pictorial representation. Before proceeding to all that, though, I need to present some important background material relating to the contents that pictures possess and to our understandings of pictures.

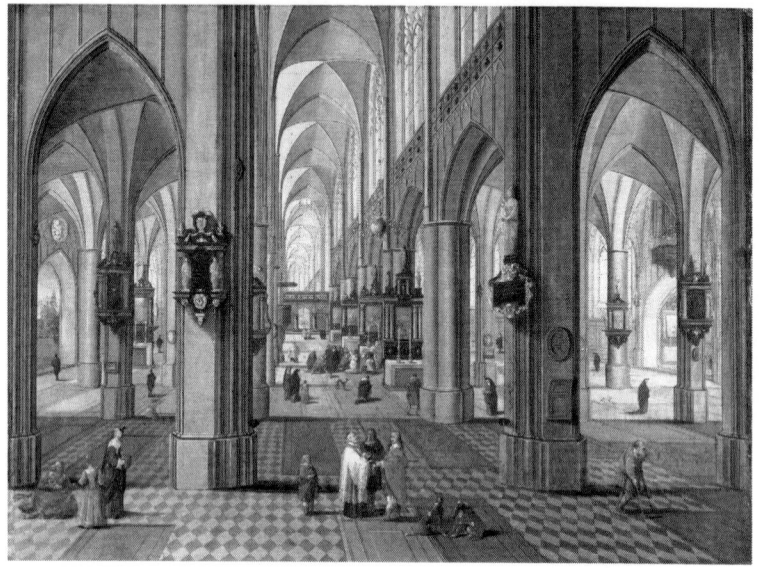

Figure 7.1. Interior of Antwerp Cathedral (*c.*1640), Pieter Neefs (the elder)[1]

Consider Figure 7.1. Figure 7.1 uses a range of pictorial techniques that have commonly been employed by Western artists since the Renaissance: the lines on the picture surface that display receding parallel lines converge upon a single area of the image's surface; and the portions of the picture that show objects diminish regularly in size as the shown items recede into the space shown by the picture. Those methods provide particularly effective tools for capturing the spatial layout of the world in relation to a single place.[2]

---

[1] © Victoria and Albert Museum, London.

[2] The spatial 'fixedness' of pictures like Figure 7.1 is explicitly reflected in some of the well-known heuristic methods for producing pictures using linear perspective and foreshortening; see, for example, the discussions in the first book of Alberti [1435–6] 1966 or the famous pair of woodcuts which Dürer produced for his 1525 *Treatise on Measurement*, showing a man drawing a reclining woman and a pair of men plotting a drawing of a foreshortened lute. Other ways of representing space in pictures have very different effects. It has seemed to many that, for instance, the representations of scenes supplied by pictures using the 'oblique' perspective commonly found in Oriental, Indian, and Persian pictures—in which receding parallel lines are depicted using lines that are themselves parallel—often involves 'not . . . a single fixed or momentary viewpoint but . . . many viewpoints', so that the process of viewing the pictures is notably reminiscent of 'our physical experience of moving through the world' and visually inspecting its contents (Hockney 2006, 204). (The remarked mobility is

Figure 7.1 does not just show things as looking one way from a unique perspective, though, even if it does capture ways that things look from one place. As one fixes one's gaze upon the bit of the picture which shows the very back of the cathedral, for instance, one grasps how things look from a perspective whose group of labelled axes labels a particular direction through the perspective's origin as *directly-forwards*. But if one's gaze is fixed upon a segment of the picture which shows one of the closest pillars, one grasps how things look from a perspective which has the same spatiotemporal origin but whose group of labelled axes incorporates a different *directly-forwards* direction.[3] The picture's distinctively visual content is therefore richly multiperspectival; and its distinctively visual content involves a corresponding multiplicity of ways for things to look.

More generally, distinctively visual pictures do not usually show things as looking just one way from a single perspective. When we comprehendingly view a picture, we normally let our eyes roam over its surface. The different views of the picture which we thereby enjoy typically disclose to us different ways that the picture shows things as looking. And there are also generally corresponding shifts in the perspectives from which the picture shows things as looking those different ways. Distinctively visual pictures thus standardly show scenes to us by showing things as looking lots of different ways from lots of different perspectives, in a fashion that exploits their own status as objects of visual investigation.

It is therefore no wonder that the process of exploring distinctively visual pictures with our eyes is apt to seem to us somewhat akin to the process of visually investigating the world. When you actually look around you, the different ways that things look to you provide you with an

---

particularly striking for certain sorts of cases in which oblique projection is customarily employed, like Chinese scroll paintings.) Arnheim says that the use of oblique projection 'conveys the sense of a world that does not confront us at a stable location but moves past us like a train' (Arnheim 1974, 280)—although it seems strange that he should assign the motion to the world.

[3] The above points may be phrased more accurately using references to the admissibility requirements included in the distinctively visual content of Figure 7.1, as discussed in Chapter 4: the admissibility requirements require that a sequence of perspective-denoting contents may fill the gaps in Figure 7.1's distinctively visual content only if, first, the perspectives denoted by the contents share a single spatiotemporal origin and, second, the labelled axes included within the perspectives denoted by the contents stand in certain systematic relations.

evolving awareness of your current environment, as the ways that things look to you reflect the ways that things actually look from numerous different visual perspectives. Likewise, when you use your eyes to explore Figure 7.1, say, the different ways that you thereby grasp the picture to show things as looking provide you with an evolving awareness of the pictured environment, as the various ways that you take the picture to shows things as looking reflect the various ways that the picture actually shows things as looking from numerous different perspectives.

Lifelikeness: locating the phenomena

Distinctively visual pictures—'pictures' *tout court*, for the rest of this chapter—often differ from one another with regard to their lifelikeness. Colour photographs showing clear views of the Eiffel Tower are more lifelike than sketchy pencil drawings of the same construction; and Vermeer's paintings of domestic interiors are more lifelike than Giotto's frescoes.

When we look comprehendingly at lifelike pictures, we acquire relatively rich senses of what it would really be like for things to look to us the ways that the pictures show things as looking. Indeed, upon reaching its limit lifelikeness results in *trompe l'œil* pictures: ones which make it seem to appropriately situated viewers that they are actually seeing things of the very sorts that the pictures show. More generally, it is natural to think that the degree of lifelikeness which belongs to a picture derives from the extent to which there is a suitable match between the look of the picture itself and the ways that it shows things as looking. (So, Sartwell speaks of the 'pre-analytic' view that 'a picture is realistic in virtue of looking like what it is a picture of'.[4])

Lifelikeness is one of the properties sometimes ascribed by saying that a picture is 'realistic'. But a survey of writing about pictures swiftly reveals that the claim that one picture is more 'realistic' than another need not amount to the claim that the first is more lifelike than the second. Walton remarks, for example, that '[s]ome kinds of realism consist in correspondences between [pictured scenes] and the actual world. The more "similar" the [pictured scene] is to the real world, the more realistic it may be said

---

[4] Sartwell 1994, 2.

to be.'[5] That last conception of realism is certainly not the same as the notion of lifelikeness. Some of Magritte's paintings are very lifelike, for example, even though they do not show the sorts of scenes which one would ever actually encounter.

Note that the intuitive thought that lifelikeness involves facts about what pictures look like does not imply that each and every possible view of a picture is relevant to its lifelikeness. Suppose, for example, that there could be some spectacles which were capable of making Vermeer's paintings look Giotto-esque. It is obvious that the possibility of those glasses does not undermine the claim that Vermeer's pictures are more lifelike than Giotto's. For we appreciate that the degree of lifelikeness which belongs to Vermeer's paintings does not depend upon how those pictures look under every set of conditions whatsoever. Rather, it depends upon how they look under a restricted range of viewing conditions which we can call the *lifelikeness-relevant* viewing conditions that are associated with the relevant pictures.

To count as lifelikeness-relevant in relation to a given picture, viewing conditions generally have to meet constraints relating to both environmental factors and the visual apparatus of the viewer. The look of a picture under ultraviolet light is rarely relevant to its lifelikeness, for instance; and the lifelikeness of a picture is not usually affected by how it looks to viewers with bad cataracts in both eyes. But the lifelikeness-relevant viewing conditions that are associated with one picture may nonetheless be quite different from those which are associated with another. The viewing conditions which are relevant to assessing the lifelikeness of, say, a ceiling fresco are generally very different to those which are relevant to determining whether a small oil painting is lifelike.[6]

Throughout the following discussion of lifelikeness, the reader should assume that whenever I speak of 'views' of a picture, or of how a picture 'looks', I am talking about views of the picture under lifelikeness-relevant viewing conditions.

---

[5] Walton 1990, 328. See also Hyman 2006, 25–7, and Lopes 1995, 277, for identification of some of the different ways in which the notion of 'realism' may be understood in relation to pictures.

[6] It is an interesting empirical question what determines the precise range of lifelikeness-relevant viewing conditions that are associated with a given picture. Some factors that are often relevant: the intentions of the picture's manufacturer, societal conventions with regard to how pictures of various sorts are to be viewed, the planned location of a picture . . .

Towards an account of lifelikeness

Figure 7.2 reproduces a cover for a cushion. Consider the representation of some poppy pods in the bottom right-hand section of that image. When one views some portion of that pod-showing bit of Figure 7.2, one grasps that the relevant picture-portion—let's call it *Pod-bit*—is showing things as looking a certain way. Let *Pod View* be that way for things to look.

Although *Pod-bit* is itself tonally very simple it does not therefore show some poppy pods whose surfaces are tonally wholly undifferentiated. Rather, *Pod-bit*'s flat tonal patterning leaves unsettled the precise nature of the tonal contrasts found over the surfaces of the pods which it shows. To revisit some ideas already encountered in Chapter 4, different possible *Pod View*-sensations differ over the range of tonal contrasts which look to be present across the surfaces of the poppy pods apparently seen in the course of those sensations. The appearance-content of *Pod View*—the common way that things look to be to the subjects of *Pod View*-

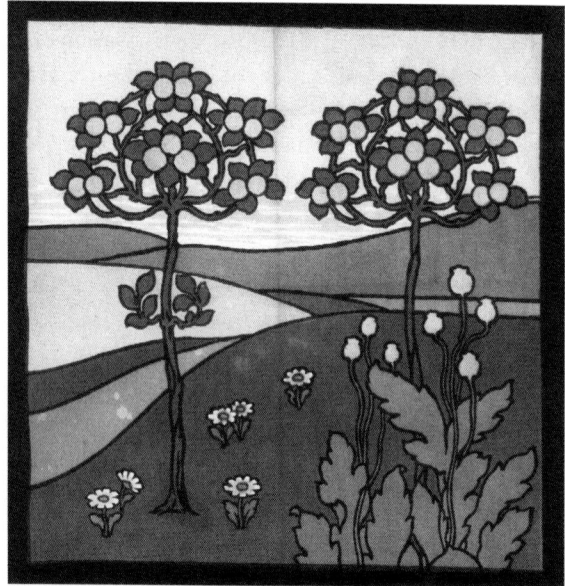

Figure 7.2. Cushion cover panel (1904), The Silver Studio (designer)[7]

[7] © Victoria and Albert Museum, London.

sensations—is therefore highly schematic; with the result that *Pod-bit* is neutral with regard to many of the features of the poppy pods which it shows.

Figure 7.2, and *Pod-bit* in particular, is not very lifelike. One natural way of elaborating that point is by noting that things can look the way that *Pod-bit* shows them as looking without their looking very much like *Pod-bit* itself looks. More precisely, consider an arbitrary view of *Pod-bit*. Consider, too, an arbitrary *Pod View*-sensation. Certain parts of the way that things look to be in the course of the first of those visual sensations will be shared by the way that things look to be in the second visual sensation. Both of the visual sensations will involve apparent confrontations with items possessing certain overall outlines, for example.

But there are very few other notable common ways that things are guaranteed to look to be in the course of our pair of arbitrary visual sensations. *Pod View*-sensations may differ from one another with regard to the tonal features of the apparently viewed poppy pods, for example. Yet views of *Pod-bit* involve apparent confrontations with 'pod outlines' that are, within their boundaries, tonally uniform.

More generally, there is a range of common features which is such that, for any possible visual sensation which is either a view of *Pod-bit* or a *Pod View*-sensation, those features are posited by the visual appearances which accompany the sensation. But that range of features is not very significant: the relevant common features do not ensure that the particular ways that things look to be in any two possible sensations of the sorts currently being considered will resemble one another significantly. There is therefore a sense in which the look of *Pod-bit* matches the way that it shows things as looking rather badly.

Now compare Figure 7.2 to Figure 7.3. Consider some part of the representation of a striped tulip on Figure 7.3's right-hand side. The way that the relevant portion of Figure 7.3—let's call it *Tulip-bit*—shows things as looking is much richer than the way that *Pod-bit* shows things as looking. In particular, there is much less variation in the different ways that things may look to be in sensations in which things look the way that *Tulip-bit* shows them as looking than there is in the visual appearances which may accompany sensations in which things look the way that *Pod-bit* shows them as looking.

Consider, for example, some possible sensation in which things look the way that *Tulip-bit* shows things as looking. We can be assured of many facts

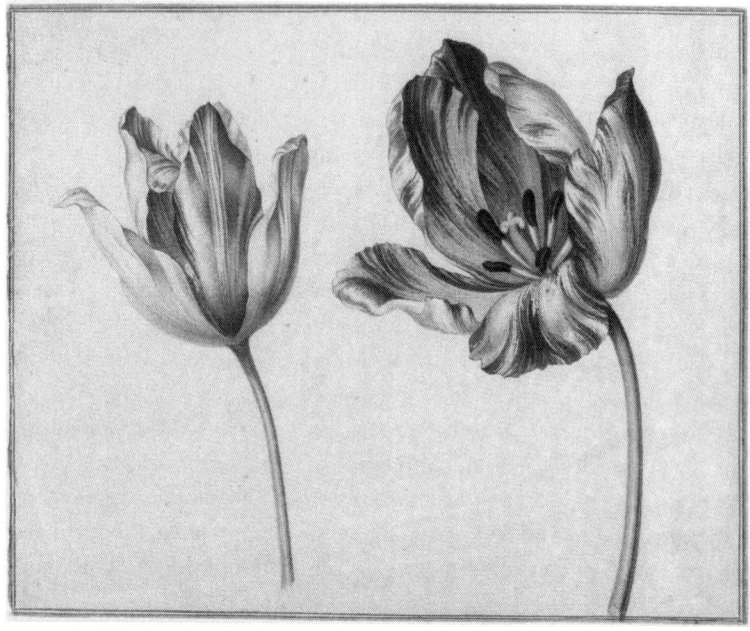

Figure 7.3. Watercolour—Tulips (after 1668), Simon (Pieterz.) Verelst[8]

about the nature of the tonal contrasts found upon the surface of the tulip that is thereby apparently seen. More generally, *Tulip-bit* provides a less schematic body of information about the striped tulip which it shows than *Pod-bit* provides about the poppy pods which it shows. *Tulip-bit* is also much more lifelike than *Pod-bit*. While looking at *Tulip-bit* is hardly exactly like looking at a striped tulip, looking at *Tulip-bit* is a lot more like looking at a striped tulip than looking at *Pod-bit* is like looking at some poppy pods.

Again, we can recast all of those points more precisely, by referring to the specifics of suitable distinctively visual contents. Let *Tulip View* be the way that *Tulip-bit* shows things as looking. The shared way that things must look to be in *Tulip View*-sensations has a relatively impressive range of features in common with the different particular ways that things may look to be in those sensations. *Tulip View*'s appearance-content is consequently less schematic than *Pod View*'s appearance-content. Hence *Tulip-bit* provides us with a much less abstract body of information about what it shows than *Pod-bit* provides us with concerning what it shows.

Consider, next, the fact that *Tulip-bit* is more lifelike than *Pod-bit*. That fact evidently corresponds to various further visible contrasts of detail between *Pod-bit* and *Tulip-bit*. The Silver Studio designers do little to model the surface of the shown poppy pods, for example, whereas Verelst uses tonal contrasts to model the receding curved surfaces of the tulip which his watercolour shows.

Those differences mean that, in comparison to *Pod-bit* and *Pod View*, the way that things look to be in any specific possible *Tulip View*-sensation will be relatively similar to the way that things look to be in any possible view of *Tulip-bit*. The visual appearances accompanying any possible view of *Tulip-bit* will resemble those accompanying any *Tulip View*-sensation in that they both posit the presence of something having a certain overall outline, for instance. But they will also resemble one another in that they both involve the apparent instantiation of a common pattern of tonal contrasts within the relevant outline. There is, as a result, quite a good match between how *Tulip-bit* looks and the ways that it shows things as looking.

The lifelikeness of Figure 7.3 as a whole is owed, though, to the fact that the viewable portions of the picture—the portions that may be unified objects of visual awareness for us (rather than, say, any portions that result from compounding scattered bits of the picture that we cannot view all at once[9])—tend to be like *Tulip-bit* in the respects just noted. But things are very different for Figure 7.2, which means that the Silver Studio design is much less lifelike than Verelst's watercolour. The degrees of lifelikeness belonging to Figures 7.2 and 7.3 in their entireties thus derive from the extent that there tends to be a certain sort of match between the looks of the viewable portions of those pictures and the ways that the relevant portions show things as looking.[10]

---

[9] Many thanks to an anonymous referee for emphasizing the need for a restriction to viewable portions of pictures here.

[10] Note that there is nothing in the above comments which requires that the resemblances being remarked should play any particular role in enabling us to grasp the distinctively visual contents of the pictures being discussed. The current approach to lifelikeness therefore chimes with an idea which has surfaced repeatedly in the recent literature, namely that theories of aspects of pictorial realism should be independent of philosophical ideas concerning the bases of depiction (see, for example, Lopes 1995, 278; and Abell 2007, 4).

An account of lifelikeness

Suppose that there is a certain range of common features which are posited by the visual appearances involved in all those possible visual sensations which are either views of a certain viewable picture-portion or visual sensations in which things look as the picture-portion shows them as looking. The *significance* of that range of common features is a measure of the extent to which their recurrence means that, for any possible view of the picture-portion and for any possible visual sensation in which things look as the picture-portion shows them as looking, there is a significant amount of resemblance between the ways that things look to be in those visual sensations.

Let's also say that *the look of* a certain viewable picture-portion *matches* the way that the picture-portion shows things as looking to the extent that the following counts as significant: the range of common features that are posited by the visual appearances involved in any possible visual sensation which is either a view of the picture-portion or a visual sensation in which things look as the picture-portion shows them as looking. Then, for instance, we saw in the previous section that the look of *Tulip-bit* matches the way that *Tulip-bit* shows things as looking—that is, *Tulip View*—to a relatively high degree. By contrast, the look of *Pod-bit* matches the way that *Pod-bit* shows things as looking—that is, *Pod View*—to a much lower degree.

The notion of a 'match' just introduced rests upon the thought that resemblances between visual appearances may be more or less 'significant'. But what exactly determines the significance of the similarities between, say, the way that things look to be in an arbitrary view of *Tulip-bit* and the ways that things look to be in an arbitrary *Tulip View*-sensation? There are various detailed answers to that question which are compatible with everything that follows, and the specifics of the correct answer largely do not matter for my purposes; the arguments below will solely rely upon a couple of very general features of the idea that the relevant sort of resemblances may be more or less significant.[11]

---

[11] In this respect, the relationship between the arguments which follow and the notion of more or less significant resemblances is similar to the relationship between, say, many arguments concerning the logical properties of counterfactual conditionals and the similarity metric upon possible worlds which is commonly used in providing a semantics for those conditionals (see, for example, Lewis 1973). For, in both cases, the relevant reasoning merely

So, to take a cue from Abell's discussion of realism, perhaps the relevant notion of significance is viewer-relative, partly depending upon the degree to which the commonalities involve the apparent presence of features which are 'relevant'[12] to a specific viewer of *Tulip-bit*. Or, to take a hint from Kulvicki's account of 'pictorial realism as a kind of verity', maybe the significance of the resemblances partly depends upon the extent to which they involve the apparent presence of features that are included 'in the observer's perceptual conception' of striped tulips.[13] But one general structural feature of the notion of significance will be crucial to some of what follows.

The look of *Tulip-bit* matches *Tulip View* to a fairly high degree. That is, for any possible view of *Tulip-bit* and for any possible *Tulip View*-sensation, there is a significant level of resemblance between the ways that things look to be in those sensations, on account of the recurrence of certain features within the contents of the visual appearances accompanying any possible sensations of the relevant kinds. But one must not underestimate the resemblance-making power of those match-making features. In particular, they allow us to see that the relatively unschematic nature of *Tulip View*'s appearance-content is no surprise.

The match-making features just considered are to be found in the contents of the visual appearances accompanying any possible visual sensation which is either a view of *Tulip-bit* or a *Tulip View*-sensation. So they are, more specifically, to be found in the contents of the visual appearances figuring in any possible *Tulip View*-sensation. But their recurrence throughout the contents of those last visual appearances means there is a significant common core running through the many specific ways that

draws upon certain very general properties of the relevant concept, meaning that the arguments can be pressed from a position of relative neutrality with regard to exactly how it ought best to be understood.

[12] Abell 2007, 12; the pertinent notion of relevance—information which 'connect[s] with viewers' existent assumptions to yield positive cognitive effects that warrant the processing effort required to obtain them'—is owed to Sperber and Wilson.

[13] Kulvicki 2006, 218. Sartwell states, similarly, that '*a picture is realistic to the extent that its visually discernible, variable properties overlap with the recognitionally relevant properties of its object*' (1994, 8). The quoted remark is an elaboration of Sartwell's more general account of realism: '[g]iven that a picture *p* represents an object *o*, *p* represents *o* realistically to the extent that *p* resembles *o* in relevant respects' (1994, 7). Sartwell's view of realism clearly has some affinities with the approach being developed in the text; Sartwell also offers some nice reflections on the aesthetic value of lifelikeness (1994, 10–11).

things may look to be in the course of *Tulip View*-sensations; that is, their recurrence means that *Tulip View*'s appearance-content is fairly unschematic.[14] More generally, we have the following:

> (7.A)   A high degree of match between the look of some picture-portion and the way that the picture-portion shows things as looking ensures that the appearance-content belonging to the latter is relatively unschematic.

With all that background in place, the previous section's discussion of Figures 7.2 and 7.3 suggest the following account of levels of lifelikeness for pictures as a whole:

> (7.B)   A picture is lifelike to the extent that the look of each of the picture's viewable portions tends to match the way that the relevant picture-portion shows things as looking.[15]

And here, for the record, is a related principle relating to unqualified lifelikeness which will be invoked at a few points below:

> (7.C)   A picture is lifelike just in case the look of each of the picture's viewable portions does indeed tend to match to a high degree the way that the relevant picture-portion shows things as looking.

Note that (7.C) is meant to be compatible with a range of different theoretical stances which may be taken in relation to out-and-out

---

[14] The inference being employed here is not trivial. The statement that the look of a picture-portion matches to a significant degree the way that it shows things as looking amounts to the claim that there is a 'relatively high degree of resemblance' between an arbitrary instance of one type and an arbitrary instance of another type. But claims of that last sort do not always imply that there is a 'relatively high degree of resemblance' between arbitrary instances of just one of the relevant types. For the standards of similarity operative within a particular context are generally informed by the particular domains of comparison at issue: what makes for a high level of resemblance when one is considering apples alone may be different to what makes for a high level of resemblance when one is considering apples and pears. The standards of similarity that are at work within two contexts may be linked, however, and the discussion in the text relies upon the thought that in the current circumstances suitable bonds are present.

[15] Distinctively visual pictures may incorporate portions which do not show things as looking certain ways. Does the presence within a distinctively visual picture of portions of the latter sort automatically reduce its lifelikeness? As it stands, principle (7.B) does not really settle that question; but the principle could be further elaborated so that the answer goes either way. The question's answer is irrelevant to what follows, however.

lifelikeness. It may be, for instance, that what counts as a 'high' degree of match varies between different contexts. If that is correct, (7.C) should be read as involving suitable context-relativizing clauses, so that the principle implies that facts about lifelikeness *simpliciter* are contextually variable too.

Some initial remarks

It was earlier remarked that lifelikeness, when taken to its extreme, results in *trompe l'œil* pictures. As an initial illustration of the explanatory powers of the preceding section's account of lifelikeness, I shall quickly demonstrate how we can explain that fact using the account. Following on from that, I will explain another equally obvious point, one about the limits of pictorial lifelikeness.

Suppose, for example, that someone produces a maximally lifelike picture that shows a pipe. Assume, more fully, that the picture shows a pipe because some portion of it—*Pipe-bit*, let's say—shows things as looking a certain way—*Pipe View*—from a perspective. *Scene-showing corresponds to seeming*: hence part of what it is for a subject to have a *Pipe View*-sensation is for the subject apparently to see a pipe.

Now, our picture is maximally lifelike. Hence in particular, and given the ideas about lifelikeness articulated previously, the look of *Pipe-bit* matches to the greatest extent the way that it shows things as looking; the look of *Pipe-bit* matches *Pipe View* to the highest degree. The range of common features which are jointly posited by the visual appearances featuring in any possible visual sensation that is either a view of *Pipe-bit* or a *Pipe View*-sensation must therefore be as significant as any such range of common features can be. The relevant range of common features must thus ensure that the way that things look to be in an arbitrary view of *Pipe-bit* resembles to the highest degree the way that things look to be in an arbitrary *Pipe View*-sensation.

Anyone who has a *Pipe View*-sensation apparently sees a pipe. But that aspect of the way that things look to be in *Pipe View*-sensations will be shared by the way that things look to be in views of *Pipe-bit*. For how, otherwise, could the way that things look to be in an arbitrary view of *Pipe-bit* resemble to the highest degree the way that things look to be in an arbitrary *Pipe View*-sensation? Hence any view of *Pipe-bit* will involve an apparent visual encounter with a pipe; that is, viewers of *Pipe-bit* will suffer from the illusion that they are seeing a pipe. Our picture is therefore a *trompe l'œil* representation of a pipe.

The earlier account of lifelikeness also easily explains some of the obvious limits to which pictorial lifelikeness tends to be subject.

Consider, for example, a photo showing a downwards-plunging view from the top of the Grand Canyon. Many of the ways that the photo shows things as looking will involve vertiginous drops through space. More precisely, given that *scene-showing corresponds to seeing*, the photo's distinctively visual content features various visual sensation-types whose appearance-contents posit deep receding spaces. Consider some such way that the picture shows things as looking—call it *Steep Drop View*—where the particular picture-portion which shows things as looking that way is *Steep Drop-bit*.

Given that *Steep Drop View*'s appearance-content is as just described, any possible *Steep Drop View*-sensation is one in which a deep receding space is apparently encountered. But, ordinarily anyway, even the most lifelike photos look fairly flat. So possible views of *Steep Drop-bit* will not similarly involve apparent encounters with steep drops. The extent to which the look of *Steep Drop-bit* matches the way that it shows things as looking—*Steep Drop View*—will therefore inevitably be non-maximal. For there will be some features which are common to all of the particular ways that things may look to be in possible *Steep Drop View*-sensations which are not also common to all of the particular ways that things may look to be in views of *Steep Drop-bit*.

More generally, then, the above account of lifelikeness straightforwardly explains why the visually apparent flatness of typical pictures means that those pictures which show deep spaces will tend never to be lifelike to the highest degree. Note, though, that if there could be pictures which themselves led viewers apparently to experience great depth— sufficiently impressive cases of stereoscopic images, perhaps[16]—the reasoning just rehearsed would not apply to them; as indeed it should not. For, just intuitively, such pictures would be able to show deep spaces in a lifelike manner, because the apparent experiences of depth to which

---

[16] Casati considers 'hallucinatory pictures', a hypothetical category of cases to which stereoscopic pictures stand in interesting relations (2010, 367); his paper focuses on the question whether 'hallucinatory pictures' ought really to be categorized as pictures. (Many thanks to an anonymous referee for the Casati reference.)

they would give rise might chime with aspects of the ways that the pictures show things as looking.

We have just seen how the ideas about lifelikeness embodied by principles (7.A)–(7.C), according to which facts about lifelikeness derive from interactions between the ways that pictures themselves look and the ways that they show things as looking, generate elegant explanations of some fundamental facts about lifelike pictures. The next couple of sections use the earlier ideas to examine some further lifelikeness-related phenomena.

Wollheim on lifelikeness

Wollheim identifies an 'elusive but noteworthy property... which we may call, interchangeably... naturalism, realism, lifelikeness, truth to nature'; a 'property [that] is identified partly by reference to a certain effect that is brought about in the spectator, and partly by reference to the way in which the picture brings about this effect'.[17] It seems clear enough from all this, and from the rest of what Wollheim says, that the property to which he refers and for which he favours the term 'naturalism', is lifelikeness.

Wollheim criticizes most previous writers on lifelikeness for tending 'to identify the naturalistic effect with the facility, or the speed, or with the irresistibility' with which we recognize what it is that a picture shows, and thereby ignoring the importance of 'our awareness of the marked surface itself'.[18] For, he says, 'the naturalistic effect comes about through a reciprocity, a particular kind of reciprocity, between the two aspects of the visual experience that we have in front of those pictures which we therefore think of as realistic'[19]—a reciprocity, as Wollheim believes, between our recognition of the contents of those pictures and our awareness of the pictures as marked surfaces.

Wollheim's talk of a 'reciprocity' captures one of the most obvious intuitive ideas about lifelikeness, the thought that lifelikeness involves a certain sort of match between the look of a picture and how it shows things as looking. But Wollheim's insistence that an awareness of lifelike pictures as marked surfaces is inevitably a factor in their special effect is unfortunate. For it implies—to my mind, counter-intuitively—that there cannot be *trompe l'œil* pictures whose production of the 'naturalistic effect'

[17] Wollheim 1987, 72.   [18] Wollheim 1987, 73.   [19] Wollheim 1987, 73.

reaches its apogee in episodes featuring visual illusions, episodes whose illusory character is partly determined by the fact that the pictures do not look to be marked surfaces to the relevant viewers.[20] The account of lifelikeness presented earlier does not share that implication.

Wollheim's stress upon the 'naturalistic effect' directs our attention to another significant aspect of lifelikeness: the degree to which a picture is lifelike relates crucially to its capacity to provoke experiences of a distinctive sort in suitable circumstances. (Budd talks, in a similar vein, of 'the experience of seeing a picture as a naturalistic depiction'.[21]) One's assessment that, say, the image of some tulips reproduced as Figure 7.3 is pretty lifelike is informed by one's sense that the picture is ripe for being experienced *as lifelike*; by one's sense that comprehending viewers of the picture will tend to recognize that there is a special harmony between the looks of the picture's viewable portions and the ways that the portions show things as looking.

Adequate accounts of lifelikeness should say something convincing about the nature of the 'naturalistic effect'. They should also provide some explanation of how the effect tends to arise. And we can use the account of lifelikeness developed earlier to do both those things. Suppose, for instance, that somebody were to produce a lifelike picture of, say, a cigar. Reconsider (7.C) above:

(7.C)   A picture is lifelike just in case the look of each of the picture's viewable portions does indeed tend to match to a high degree the way that the relevant picture-portion shows things as looking.

[20] Wollheim 1987, 62. Wollheim's views on the nature of reciprocity correspond to his view that the visual episodes in which we see things in pictures (see the next chapter for more on 'seeing-in') invariably incorporate an awareness of those pictures as marked surfaces; for criticisms of Wollheim on that score, see for instance Lopes 1996, 47–51; and Levinson 1998, 227–33. See also Casati 2010, whose hypothetical category of hallucinatory pictures is relevant here.

[21] Budd 1993, 168. Budd's account of this experience invokes his concept of the 'visual field' which forms part of a given visual episode: 'my visual field is just my visual world [—the complete way the world is represented to me by my visual experience—] considered in abstraction from one of its three spatial dimensions, namely, distance outwards from my point of view' (1993, 158). He claims that one sees a picture as a naturalistic depiction 'to the degree that there is an experienced match' between the visual field which forms part of the way that the picture looks to one and the visual field which would form part of the visual experience of someone who viewed the scene depicted by the picture (1993, 168). Budd's account of the experience of naturalism has clear affinities to the approach being developed in this chapter.

Given (7.C), the look of the picture's viewable portions tend to match to a high degree the ways that those picture-portions show things as looking.

But suppose that you view one of the picture's portions—*Cigar-bit*—where *Cigar-bit*'s look does match to a high degree the way—*Cigar View*—that it shows things as looking. By the latter condition, the contents of the visual appearances accompanying any specific possible view of *Cigar-bit* significantly resemble the contents of the visual appearances which accompany any particular possible *Cigar View*-sensation, because of certain features that look to be present in any possible sensation which is of one of those kinds. More specifically, therefore, the way that things looked to you to be in the course of your view of *Cigar-bit* significantly resembles the way that things look to be in the course of any possible *Cigar View*-sensation.

Recall, though, that *distinctively sensory showing comes from subjective informativeness*: one who grasps the distinctively visual content of our envisaged picture thereby singles out *Cigar View* in terms of the subjective character which is common to all and only the possible *Cigar View*-sensations. Your comprehending view of *Cigar-bit* therefore provided you with an appreciation of the subjective character of the common way that things look to be in the course of *Cigar View*-sensations. Hence you were likely to have been struck by the significant phenomenological consonance between the way that *Cigar-bit* actually looked to you to be and the way that you understood *Cigar-bit* to be showing things as looking. Wollheim's talk of the 'naturalistic effect' is, I conjecture, just a way of recording the fact that lifelike pictures are able to lead viewers to the sort of realization just described.

Information and lifelikeness

Lifelike pictures are sometimes particularly handy. If one wishes to find mushrooms to eat, for instance, it is useful to have access to lifelike pictures providing relatively close-up and straightforward views of mushrooms of different specified kinds. Woe betide anyone who, seeking liberty caps, feasts on destroying angels! Various philosophers have consequently sought to relate lifelikeness to certain special properties of the information which lifelike pictures provide.

Schier, for example, singles out a type of realism which may belong to a caricature while 'lacking in a spare but veridical drawing', and which seems to answer to the concept of lifelikeness; he holds that the relevant type of realism consists in 'maximal commitment' with respect to the visually recognizable properties that realistic pictures show items as having.[22] And Abell holds that '[a] picture is realistic *qua picture of an object type* to the extent that the depictive information it provides about how an object of the type it depicts would look, were one to see an object of that type, is relevant'.[23]

Abell and Schier are united in the thought that the lifelikeness of lifelike pictures consists in their possession of certain informational properties. The general idea that lifelike pictures have special informational properties seems clearly to be correct; a lifelike picture of, say, a griffin somehow 'tells us more' about the look of what it shows than does a less lifelike picture of a griffin. But might it not be that the interesting informational features of lifelike pictures are to be *explained* in terms of the more fundamental fact that lifelikeness involves suitable interactions between the ways that pictures themselves look and the ways that the pictures show things as looking?

To begin, note that the informational properties of lifelike pictures are fairly subtle. Someone might think that highly lifelike pictures will always be minutely detailed, for instance, but that is not so. Somebody could produce an extraordinarily lifelike painting of a foggy scene, say, where part of the lifelikeness of that picture would reside precisely in its encapsulation of the ways that fog erodes fine visible detail. The 'impressive detail' which lifelike pictures involve does not reduce to their telling us lots and

---

[22]   Schier 1986, 176.

[23]   Abell 2007, 11; Abell states that '[t]he most basic form of realism, realism *simpliciter*, is pictures' realism qua pictures of object type' (2007, 13), and the examples which she provides seem to indicate that this most basic form of realism is lifelikeness. (Abell's account also has another component besides the one quoted above, which is meant to capture the idea of a picture's being a realistic representation of a certain particular: '[a] picture is realistic *qua picture of a particular* to the extent that the depictive information it provides about how the particular it depicts would look, were one to see it, is relevant' (2007, 11).) Relatedly, Lopes holds that 'a picture is realistic to the extent that it belongs to an appropriately informative system', that is to a 'pictorial system' that 'makes commitments [with regard to the nature of the items depicted in pictures within the system] which satisfy requirements as to the kind of information pictures should convey for the purposes they serve in given contexts' (Lopes 1995, 283). The nature of the relationships between Lopes's notion of 'realism' and lifelikeness are not fully clear to me, however, so I have not considered his views in the text.

lots. It is, rather, a matter of their tending to provide relatively refined reflections of the details which would seem to confront those viewers to whom things really looked the ways that the pictures show things as looking.

These points are straightforwardly explicable once we assume the earlier account of lifelikeness. Consider some lifelike picture. By the principle (7.C) requoted in the previous section, the picture's lifelikeness means that the look of its viewable portions tend to match to a high degree the ways that those picture-portions show things as looking. But now consider some viewable portion of the picture which conforms to that trend. And suppose that the relevant picture-portion shows, say, a house seen in fog, where *House-in-Fog View* is the way that the picture-portion—*Fogbound House-bit*—shows things as looking. Then there is a high degree of match between the look of *Fogbound House-bit* and *House-in-Fog View*.

Reconsider principle (7.A) above:

(7.A) A high degree of match between the look of some picture-portion and the way that the picture-portion shows things as looking ensures that the appearance-content belonging to the latter is relatively unschematic.

By that principle, the appearance-content of *House-in-Fog View* is fairly unschematic; it amounts to a pretty low-level abstraction from the specific ways that things may look to be in *House-in-Fog View*-sensations.

But *scene-showing corresponds to seeming*: the information which *Fogbound House-bit* provides about what it shows is thus settled by what is included in *House-in-Fog View*'s appearance-content. Hence the information which *Fogbound House-bit* provides about the fogbound house which it shows will have a significant range of features in common with the information which any particular possible *House-in-Fog View*-sensation would provide about the nature of what is thereby apparently seen.

The details included in *Fogbound House-bit*'s showing of a house in fog are thus 'true to life' in the following sense: they overlap significantly with the visual details of a house in fog which would apparently be manifested to any viewer who had a *House-in-Fog View*-sensation. And the lifelikeness of our picture as a whole means that the information provided by its viewable portions will generally tend to be true to life in the very way that the information supplied by *Fogbound House-bit* is true to life. For the ways that those picture-portions show things as looking will tend to be relatively rich, in that their appearance-contents will be relatively unschematic.

The subjective informativeness of distinctively visual contents also brings to the fore another crucial informational aspect of lifelike pictures, one having to do with the felt character of suitable sorts of visual sensations.[24]

Suppose that one views the picture-portion *Fogbound House-bit* just discussed. *Distinctively sensory showing comes from subjective informativeness*: one's grasp of the way that *Fogbound House-bit* shows a house in fog as looking will therefore be mediated by an appreciation of what it would be like apparently to see a house in fog which looks that way. But, as just noted, *House-in-Fog View*'s appearance-content is fairly unschematic; there is a significant level of resemblance between the different ways that things may look to be in *House-in-Fog View*-sensations. One's appreciation of the subjective character which is common to all and only the possible *House-in-Fog View*-sensations will thus provide one with a fairly rich sense of what it is like to have any specific possible *House-in-Fog View*-sensation.

The previous account of lifelikeness therefore implies that comprehending views of *Fogbound House-bit*, and of picture-portions of lifelike pictures more generally, will be 'true to life' in another vital sense: they will offer us a relatively refined awareness of what things would be like for any viewer who had a specific sensation in which things look the way that the picture-portion shows things as looking. But one major aspect of our intuitive understanding of lifelikeness just is the thought that comprehending views of lifelike pictures will tend to supply us with comparatively rich senses of what it would really be like for things to look to us the ways that the pictures show things as looking. The account of lifelikeness formulated above accommodates that point.

---

[24] It is not completely clear whether the 'subjective' informational features that I am about to discuss are acknowledged by Schier's informational approach to realism; there may be some way of teasing them out of his account of realism in terms of maximal commitment along with his central idea about the nature of depiction—that facts about what pictures depict arise from their potential to engage suitably with our capacities to recognize things by sight. Abell's account—with its reliance upon the idea of information concerning how 'an object of the type [that a given picture depicts] would look' (Abell 2007, 11)—is surely meant to encompass the subjective informational features discussed in the text, however. (See, for example, her claim to have provided an account of realism which 'exploits the fact that pictures provide information about their objects' appearances' (2007, 17).)

Throughout the previous chapter, and up to this point in the current one, I have generally been studiously non-committal with regard to whether particular pictures show things as looking certain ways in the course of visual sensations or whether they just show things as looking certain ways from perspectives. And this is because nothing has hung upon the issue: the earlier account of lifelikeness applies across the board, for instance.

It seems obvious that there are pictures that show things as looking certain ways from perspectives without also showing things as looking certain ways in the course of sensations. (We generally interpret automatically taken photographs as merely showing things as looking certain ways from perspectives, for example.) But, as we will see in the next section, it also seems clear that there can be sensation-characterizing pictures; that is, it seems clear that pictures may portray visual sensations, by showing things as looking certain ways in the course of visual episodes.[25] The rest of this chapter looks at some interesting questions commonly raised by those pictures which we are inclined to construe as sensation-characterizing distinctively visual representations.

Picturing vision

Consider Figure 7.4. Le Nain's picture exhibits certain features that, to my eyes at least, make it fairly natural to regard the image as portraying a visual episode: it is tempting to take the eyes of the girl shown in the picture as meeting the gaze of an onlooker, for instance. Whether or not that interpretation of the picture is correct, though, the picture surely could have been meant to bear that sort of construal. For the sake of argument, then, let's suppose that Figure 7.4 does portray a visual sensation.

---

[25] The thought that pictures sometimes portray visual sensations is fairly common in the literature. Wollheim considers a series of pictures by Friedrich, for example, stating that 'we should think of Friedrich . . . as going from viewer to viewpoint to view. In Friedrich's work the high viewpoint is essentially occupied' (Wollheim 1987, 133; for the whole discussion of Friedrich, see Wollheim 1987, 131–40). Similarly, Koerner starts his book on Friedrich with a discussion of a painting of some 'Trees and Bushes in the Snow', saying that aspects of one's experiences in comprehendingly viewing the picture compel one to interpret the painting 'as the picture of an *experience* of a thicket' (2009, 12); more generally, he writes that 'Friedrich's landscapes present themselves as something seen, rather than simply as something there' (2009, 213).

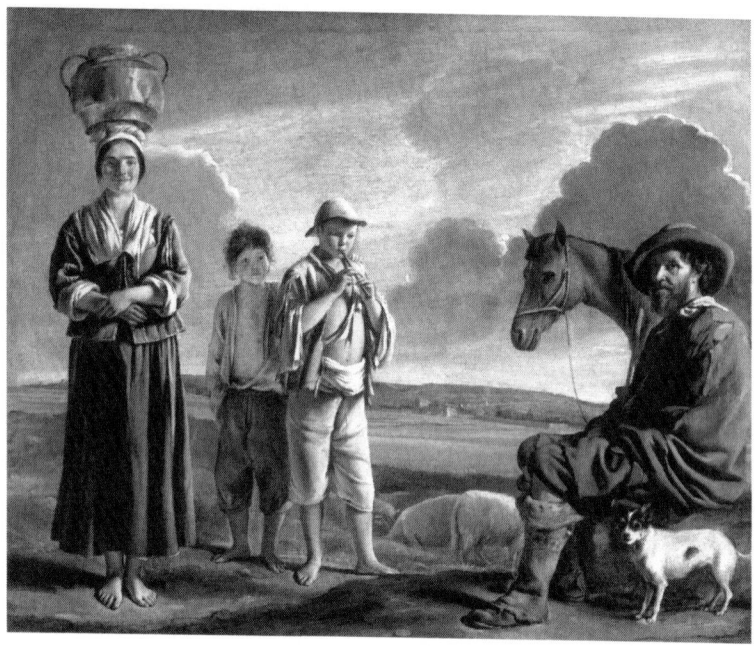

Figure 7.4. The Resting Horseman (1640s), Louis Le Nain[26]

In line with the observations at the start of this chapter, note that Figure 7.4 does not show things as looking just one way. So, look at Figure 7.4 and meet the gaze of the girl shown in the image. In so doing, you grasp that Figure 7.4 shows things as looking a certain way: *Girl's Gaze View*. Next, look again at Figure 7.4, and meet the gaze of the seated man shown in the picture. The way which you thereby grasp that Le Nain's picture shows things as looking—*Man's Gaze View*—is distinct[27] from *Girl's Gaze View*: in particular, *Man's Gaze View*-sensations focus upon a man's eyes whereas *Girl's Gaze View*-sensations focus upon a girl's eyes. Both *Girl's Gaze View* and *Man's Gaze View* seem like ideal candidates for being ways that Le Nain's picture shows things as looking in the course of a visual sensation.

---

[26] © Victoria and Albert Museum, London.

[27] That is, they are ways for things to look that do not share possible instances. This feature of the relevant ways for things to look, which I have tacitly combined with the assumption that Le Nain's painting does not portray an impossible visual sensation, is important to the arguments which follow.

Let's suppose, first, that Le Nain's picture characterizes exactly one of the numerous distinct ways that it shows things as looking as being a way that things look in the course of a visual sensation. Given that *Girl's Gaze View* and *Man's Gaze View* seem to be ideal candidates for being ways that Figure 7.4 shows things as looking in the course of visual sensations, let's suppose that Le Nain's picture portrays a visual sensation of just one of those kinds. Then the content of the picture ensures that it either portrays a *Girl's Gaze View*-sensation or a *Man's Gaze View*-sensation, but not both.

This seems silly. Although Le Nain doubtless could have meant for his picture to portray, say, a *Girl's Gaze View*-sensation rather than a *Man's Gaze View*-sensation, it is unlikely that his intentions were as definite as all that. But what else, besides Le Nain's intentions, would enable us to pick one of the ways that the picture shows things as looking, to the exclusion of all the others, as subsuming the one and only visual sensation that the painting can properly be regarded as portraying?

So let's suppose, second, that more than one of the distinct ways that Figure 7.4 shows things as looking is such that the picture shows things as looking that way in the course of a visual sensation. That supposition immediately raises questions about the relations between the times at which the image characterizes the portrayed visual sensations as occurring. Does Le Nain's picture allow for the possibility that some of those visual sensations are simultaneous, for example, or does it characterize them all as being spread out over a series of distinct moments?[28]

The first of those options—the 'permitting simultaneity' one—is bizarre. Our comprehension of Figure 7.4 certainly does not force us to accept that the painting portrays a number of distinct yet simultaneous visual sensations. The 'permitting simultaneity' option must therefore involve the thought that the picture portrays numerous visual sensations, where the picture's content leaves open both the possibility that the visual

---

[28] To put those questions more precisely, using some of the additional apparatus introduced in Chapter 4: on the approach being entertained in the text, do the admissibility requirements included in the distinctively visual content of Figure 7.4 allow the relevant gaps in the content to be completed by contents denoting simultaneous visual sensations; or do they demand that those gaps should be completed by contents denoting non-simultaneous visual sensations? There are numerous points in the following discussion at which admissibility requirements may be invoked to provide more precise accounts of certain phenomena specified in the main text.

sensations occur at the same time and also the possibility that they occur at distinct times. But that studied neutrality with regard to the temporal location of a range of distinct portrayed visual sensations surely answers to nothing that is recoverable from our comprehension of Le Nain's painting.

How about the idea that the picture portrays numerous sensations as occurring at a range of distinct times? While it does not in itself seem unnatural to interpret the picture as portraying a visual episode that is somewhat extended in time—one in which a spectator meets a girl's gaze and a seated man's gaze in quick succession, for instance—what are we then to say about the temporal order in which the portrayed sensations occur?

Assume that, say, the picture portrays a *Girl's Gaze View*-sensation as occurring at one time and a *Man's Gaze View*-sensation as occurring at another very close time. Which time comes first? There seems to be no non-arbitrary way of answering that question: there seems to be no reason for taking the picture to portray a *Girl's Gaze View*-sensation followed by a *Man's Gaze View*-sensation rather than vice versa. That point makes it very hard to see how we may coherently claim that the picture portrays non-simultaneous but temporally neighbouring sensations of each of the two stated kinds.

On the one hand, then, there does not seem to be any acceptable way of construing Le Nain's picture as characterizing just one way for things to look as being a way that things look in the course of a visual sensation. But, on the other hand, there also does not seem to be any acceptable way of interpreting Le Nain's picture as characterizing more than one way for things to look as being a way that things look in the course of a visual sensation. But if the picture portrays a visual sensation, it must surely be correctly interpretable in one of those two ways. So it seems that the picture does not portray a visual sensation after all.

Analogues of the points just made can be applied to very many pictures, to provide purported demonstrations that the pictures do not portray visual sensations.[29] They can be adapted, for example, to apply to the

---

[29] It is worth noting that the relevant points do not apply to individual visual mental images: if one produces a snapshot-like visual mental image that shows, say, a table then the visual mental image shows things as looking a single way. Note, too, that there was nothing in the foregoing which implied that there could not be pictures which, say, show how things look in the course of a multitude of simultaneous visual sensations; it is just that there do not in fact seem to be many pictures which we would happily regard as being of that sort.

pictures in comics which are sometimes used in the telling of first-person narratives, and which often seem very clearly to be meant to portray the visual sensations of their narrators. Similarly, they can be adapted to apply to passages of moving pictures, even to ones which employ some of the cinematic devices that we typically take to indicate that we are being shown how things look to someone. The preceding arguments therefore look a little too powerful to be convincing. What is to be done?

Ambiguities

Figure 7.4 shows things as looking many different ways, as noted previously. But we need not therefore assume that all of the ways that the picture shows things as looking are equally good candidates for being ways that the picture shows things as looking in the course of a visual sensation. So, focus upon the portion of Le Nain's picture that shows the rump of the closest sheep. You thereby grasp that the picture shows things as looking a certain way. It is natural to take that rather peripheral way for things to look as merely helping to characterize the scene shown by the picture.

Yet we still seem to have too many candidates for the sorts of sensations which the picture might reasonably be taken to portray. It is very hard to see how one might justify the claim that Le Nain's painting portrays a *Girl's Gaze View*-sensation rather than a *Man's Gaze View*-sensation, for example; and vice versa. Yet it is equally hard to see how one may coherently elaborate the thought that the picture portrays sensations of both those kinds. There is a way through these issues, though; and once the path is clear, we will be able to understand how it is that pictures commonly manage to portray visual sensations. For there is nothing to stop us from treating Figure 7.4 as being irresolvably *ambiguous*.

We can hold, for example, that there is an acceptable construal of Figure 7.4 on which the picture just portrays a *Girl's Gaze View*-sensation. On that reading of the image, each other way that the picture shows things as looking—including *Man's Gaze View*—is then a way that the picture shows things as looking from a perspective that is simultaneous with the portrayed sensation. But we can also say that, on another equally acceptable interpretation of Figure 7.4, the picture portrays a *Man's Gaze View*-sensation; where again, on that reading, each other way that the picture shows things as looking—including *Girl's Gaze View*—is a way that the image shows things as looking from a perspective that is simultaneous with the portrayed sensation.

Both of those readings of Le Nain's picture bind it to a single moment. The multiplicity of acceptable readings of that momentary sort mirrors the fact that, while it is fair to interpret the picture as portraying a momentary visual sensation, there is no way that the picture shows things as looking which is to be identified as the one and only way that the picture shows things as looking in the course of a visual sensation. While it seems perfectly acceptable to construe Figure 7.4 as relating to just one time, however, it does not seem to be obligatory. As noted previously, for instance, one might naturally take the image to portray a short visual episode in which a couple of gazes are met in quick succession. To make sense of that option, we may invoke a further range of equally acceptable but distinct readings of Figure 7.4.

On one acceptable reading of Le Nain's picture, for instance, it portrays a *Girl's Gaze View*-sensation that is closely followed by a *Man's Gaze View*-sensation; on that reading the picture also shows things as looking a multitude of distinct ways from perspectives that are simultaneous with the relevant sensations. But there is another acceptable construal of the picture on which it portrays a *Man's Gaze View*-sensation that is very soon followed by a *Girl's Gaze View*-sensation; on that interpretation the picture again also shows things as looking a multitude of distinct ways from perspectives that are simultaneous with the relevant sensations. Many further readings of the same temporally extended sort are available.

More generally, there are many pictures which we naturally interpret as showing how things look in the course of visual episodes. But, when we have a picture of that kind, it is standardly like Figure 7.4 in the following respects. First, there are many ways that the picture shows things as looking. Second, not all of those ways for things to look are plausibly taken to be *portrayal-eligible* relative to the picture; that is, not all of them can plausibly be viewed as ways that things look in the visual episode portrayed by the picture. Yet, third, there are still numerous ways for things to look which might reasonably be taken to be portrayal-eligible.

We can nonetheless treat the assumed picture as a sensation-characterizing distinctively visual representation, by diagnosing a serious case of ambiguity. On this approach, the portrayal-eligible ways for things to look generate a host of distinct admissible readings of the picture. The relevant readings may sometimes include ones on which the picture portrays a single visual sensation of some portrayal-eligible kind, for example; and they may sometimes include ones on which the picture portrays temporally extended sequences of visual sensations that belong to portrayal-eligible kinds. The ways that the picture shows things as looking that are not portrayal-eligible also feature in the admissible readings of the picture, though, as ways that the image shows things as looking from perspectives that are suitably related to the visual sensations that the readings characterize the picture as portraying.

It should be noted that the resulting range of pictorial interpretations is not like the various different readings which may be employed in relation to a typical utterance of, say, 'I went to the bank'. For, in that last case, circumstances—a current concern with angling, for instance—will dictate that one of readings in the range is actually better than the others. By contrast, the ambiguity in the pictorial case is 'irresolvable' in that each of the available readings is equally acceptable in the light of all further relevant facts.

I think that this is an intuitively attractive way of handling pictures like Figure 7.4. On the one hand, the idea that, say, Le Nain's painting cannot coherently be interpreted as characterizing a visual episode from the inside seems unacceptable. But, on the other, one just cannot identify a unique visual sensation, or indeed a unique sequence of successive visual sensations, which the painting might fairly be regarded as portraying; there are many ideal candidates for the job. Should we therefore say that the picture portrays lots of visual sensations that take place at the very same time? That seems ludicrous. What option remains, other than to treat the picture as being irresolvably ambiguous—as having various equally acceptable readings which differ with regards to what sort of visual episode it is that the picture is taken to portray?[30]

---

[30] The above section presented a slightly simplified version of what I am tempted to regard as the correct approach to the issues discussed. In particular, I am inclined to think that the various 'acceptable readings' of, say, Figure 7.4 are best viewed as analogues of the precisifications of vague terms posited by supervaluationist theorists of vagueness (see, for instance, Keefe 2000 for more on supervaluationism). The distinctively visual content of Le Nain's picture may then be regarded as being incomplete in a certain sense, rather than as being ambiguous. (Something like the relevant sort of incompleteness is invoked by Walton when he writes that '[c]harity may favour allowing, by default, that fictionally the spectator of [Watteau's *Embarkation for Cythera*] observes the scene in a normal manner; but there will be little to be said about the specifics, about what, fictionally, he looks at when and for how long' (Walton 1990, 327–8).)

8

Distinctively Sensory Records

The reader has no doubt once viewed a snapshot whose origins were entirely unknown to him or her. When that occurs, there is a way in which one's appreciation of the relevant photo is merely partial. For while one may grasp in the barest sense how it is that the photo shows things as looking 'from various perspectives', one knows nothing of the precise whereabouts and whenabouts of the historical perspectives whose surrounding environment the photo captures.

The notion of distinctively sensory content does not itself capture the past-directed aspects of the especially visual information which photographs may give to those in the know. For recall that distinctively sensory contents were taken in Chapter 3 to have a gappy adjectival form, precisely to mirror the fact that one may in the most basic sense understand a distinctively sensory representation without thereby linking the representation to any specific sensations or perspectives. It is thus clear that the importance which we accord to photos often derives from more than their distinctively sensory contents.

The emotional worth of family photos, for example, generally depends upon their being faithful records of things that really did happen. Yet, although we do not just want our photo albums to be filled with distinctively visual representations, the fact that they are occupied by distinctively visual representations is hardly beside the point. Can this book's theory of distinctively sensory content be used to shed light upon the various forms of significance which we typically accord to distinctively sensory representations like photographs, and to somewhat related cases like the sensory mental images often accompanying our apparent recollections of the past?

To answer that question, I will have to leave the confines of the theory, by introducing additional assumptions relating to various sorts of distinctively sensory representations. But many aspects of the earlier treatment of distinctively sensory content will be central to the resulting answers.

Indeed, the theory will be precisely what provides those answers with a nice degree of generality. The following section introduces a family of distinctively sensory representations that will be central to the rest of this chapter.

Distinctively sensory records

One important consequence of the gappy adjectival nature of distinctively sensory contents is that it enables them to feature in more complex contents.

Produce a visual mental image which shows things as looking a certain way from a perspective. You may consider the hypothesis that, for some specific perspective *a* that is near to your own current position, things look from *a* the way that the visual mental image shows things as looking. The content of that hypothesis builds upon the distinctively visual content of your visual mental image, by plugging the gap in the image's distinctively visual content using a content that denotes *a*. The hypothesis involves treating the visual mental image as not just showing how things look from 'a perspective', but as showing how things look from *a* in particular.

We tend to pick out the past perspectives that are relevant to distinctively sensory representations like photographs in a pretty rough manner, rather than by naming them. We usually just gesture at the times and places at which the origins of the perspectives were located. And doing that anyway enables us to transmit the sort of information about past perspectives which we usually wish to communicate by means of distinctively sensory representations.

Thus consider Figure 8.1. If I wanted to tell you more about the significance of this photo, I would not name the particular perspectives from which things once looked as the photo shows them as looking. I would instead provide you with information which, while being in some ways less specific, is more informative: I can tell you, for instance, that the snapshot shows how things looked from some perspectives found in Northampton during 2010.

Consider the sentence 'there was a red ball'. We may regard the content of that sentence as resulting from the use of an 'existential quantifier' (*there was a ball x such that . . .*) to fill the gaps in a gappy content (_ *was red*) using a 'bound variable' (*x*, in this case), thereby yielding the following overall:

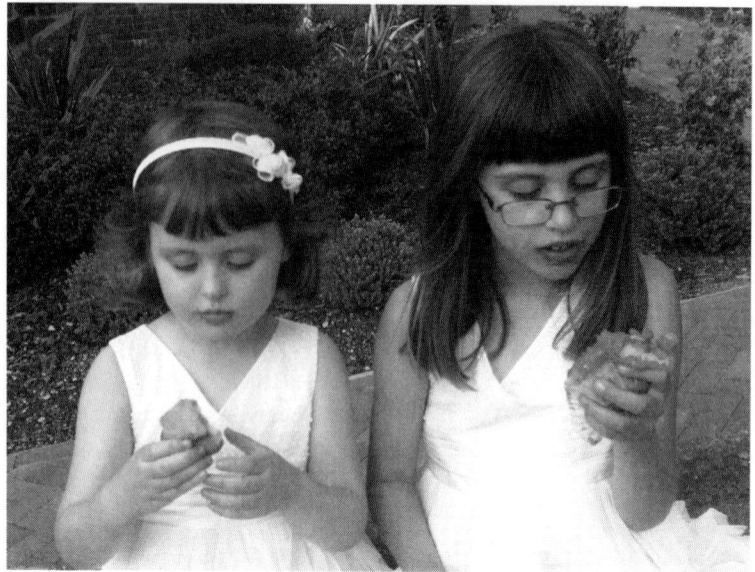

Figure 8.1. Miranda and Lydia eating cupcakes (2010), Rosanna Keefe

there was a ball x such that x was red. More generally, the gaps in gappy adjectival contents may be completed by prefixing the adjectival contents with existential quantifiers, where those last are the contents which we may express linguistically using phrases like 'there is an *x* such that' and 'some *y* was such that'. The ensuing contents then relate to groups of items in a relatively non-specific manner.[1]

I asserted earlier that Figure 8.1 shows how things looked from some perspectives found in Northampton during 2010: 'from some 2010-Northampton perspectives', for short. In making that assertion, I was presenting a certain content as true. And, in accepting my assertion, you accepted the content which I presented as true. The relevant content is a content that is constructed from the gappy distinctively visual content of Figure 8.1, in broadly the sort of manner described in the previous paragraph.

Suppose, more fully, that one simply grasps the ways that Figure 8.1 shows things as looking 'from some perspectives'. Then one associates the

---

[1] As the reader may know, there is a lot more to be said about all this—and it can be said a lot more precisely—but for our purposes the simple ideas articulated in the text will do.

picture with a certain gappy perspective-characterizing distinctively visual content. When I made my earlier assertion, I was presenting as true the content which is generated from that gappy content by prefixing it with the existential quantifier *there were some 2010-Northampton perspectives x, y, . . . such that x, y, . . .*[2] And, in accepting my assertion, you came to accept the existentially quantified past-directed content thereby generated.

For simplicity's sake, let's focus for the moment upon exclusively perspective-characterizing distinctively sensory representations: those that just show things as standing sensorily certain ways from perspectives, rather than in the course of sensations. Extrapolating from the above discussion of Figure 8.1, suppose that we are given an exclusively perspective-characterizing distinctively sensory representation. Numerous contents may be based upon the representation's distinctively sensory content, by plugging the content's gaps using existential quantifiers ranging over domains of historic perspectives. The resulting contents are past-directed, in that they concern the ways that things once stood sensorily from perspectives to be found within appropriate domains of past perspectives.[3]

Figure 8.1 actually does show how things looked from some 2010-Northampton perspectives. It is therefore a 'distinctively sensory record' in relation to the domain of 2010-Northampton perspectives. More generally, suppose that we are given a distinctively sensory representation. And suppose that some existentially quantified past-directed content built upon the representation's distinctively sensory content is true, a past-directed

---

[2] This simplifies things a bit, by ignoring the fact that Figure 8.1 shows how things looked from a range of past perspectives that stand in certain crucial relationships to one another, relationships that are captured by the admissibility requirements that form part of Figure 8.1's distinctively visual content (see Chapter 4 for more discussion of admissibility requirements). (Figure 8.1 shows how things looked from a group of past perspectives that are located at a single place at a single time, but which differ from one another in certain systematic ways with regards to the groups of labelled axes which they contain, as explained at the start of Chapter 7.) The existential quantifier that is prefixed to the distinctively visual content belonging to Figure 8.1, to yield the past-directed content that I presented as true in the course of my earlier assertion, should therefore really be taken to amount to something like the following: *there were some 2010-Northampton perspectives x, y, . . . satisfying the admissibility requirements C such that x, y, . . .* I have ignored these sorts of issues in the main text, however, to avoid additional clutter.

[3] Suppose that the distinctively visual content of Figure 8.1 is non-conceptual, in one or more of the senses distinguished in Chapter 4. Are any of the existentially quantified past-directed contents which may be based upon the distinctively visual content of Figure 8.1 also non-conceptual in the relevant senses? That is an interesting question, but it is not one on which I will take a stand here.

content whose existential quantifiers range over a certain domain D of historic perspectives. Then the distinctively sensory representation is a *distinctively sensory record* in relation to D.

We commonly regard photographs as being distinctively sensory records in relation to domains of past perspectives. We also often regard playbacks of audio recordings and of films as being distinctively sensory records in relation to domains of past perspectives. Or consider the sensory mental images by means of which we apparently recall our own pasts; the *apparently recollective* sensory mental images which occur in *apparent sensory memories*. We commonly take apparently recollective sensory mental images to be distinctively sensory records in relation to domains of past perspectives that stood in appropriate spatiotemporal relationships to events from our own pasts.

The notion of distinctively sensory content, by providing the foundation for an explication of the notion of a distinctively sensory record, thus helps us to bring under one heading a diverse range of cases which can connect us to the past in a notable manner and in which distinctively sensory representations play a central role.

Distinctively sensory record⋆s

The conditions which a distinctively sensory representation must meet to count as a distinctively sensory record are pretty demanding. In fact, they are demanding enough that they are not met by some of the most obvious and interesting types of cases in which distinctively sensory representations link us to the past.

Reconsider the drawing by Watteau reproduced in Chapter 4, as Figure 4.5. Let's suppose, just for the sake of an example, that Watteau's drawing is a portrait of someone. According to the previous section, the picture is a distinctively sensory record in relation to the domain *early rococo* of late seventeenth- to early eighteenth-century French perspectives just in case each way that the image shows things as looking is a way that things looked from an *early rococo* perspective.

But Watteau's picture therefore probably is not a distinctively sensory record in relation to the *early rococo* perspectives. For one thing, Watteau doubtless paid more attention to getting right some parts of the drawing's subject than others: he may not have troubled himself greatly with the bits of the picture depicting the subject's left thigh, for instance. And there may be some of the parts of the drawing that were not even intended to reflect ways that things looked from perspectives near to the picture's subject; perhaps Watteau filled them in at a later date. Hence there may well be ways that the picture shows things as looking which were not ways that things looked from any *early rococo* perspectives.

More importantly, though, handmade portraits like Watteau's drawing are the results of extended periods of studying their subjects. And it is, I suspect, a rare portraitist whose portraits are meant to show how their subjects looked at some specific moment during the subject's sitting. Accordingly, the documentary interest of handmade portraits does not derive from their being distinctively sensory records as defined above. It is, instead, owed to their satisfaction of conditions that are a little harder to pin down; we tend to take accurate handmade portraits to capture the gist of a sitter's visual appearance at some time.

Those sorts of considerations do not apply to handmade portraits alone. In particular, while apparently recollective sensory mental images some- times strike us as being stereotypically photo-like, they surely also often seem to us rather to be portrait-like. That is, we commonly regard the memorial status of the images as being compatible with their failing to capture *exactly* how things stood sensorily from any of the perspectives to be found during the recalled period. Instead, we take it that the images merely capture *pretty much* how things once stood sensorily from some of the relevant perspectives.[4] How far do those last points and the others made earlier in this section limit the interest of the remaining parts of this chapter?

Not much. Let's say that an exclusively perspective-characterizing distinctively sensory representation is a *distinctively sensory record** in relation to a domain D of historic perspectives, relative to a certain portion P of the representation's distinctively sensory content, just in case the ways for things to stand sensorily figuring in P are suitably similar to ways that things stood sensorily from some perspectives in D. (What counts as 'suitable similarity' will be fixed by some contextually determined standards.) That is, let's say that an exclusively perspective-characterizing distinctively sensory

---

[4] Many thanks to Rosanna Keefe for impressing this point upon me and for emphasizing that I had tended to overestimate the extent of the class of putative distinctively sensory records.

representation is a distinctively sensory record★ in relation to D, relative to P, just in case the content generated by prefixing the specific portion P with the existential quantifier *there were some perspectives x, y, . . . in D such that, pretty much,* _ is actually true.[5]

It may well be, for instance, that Watteau's Figure 4.5 is not a distinctively sensory record in relation to the *early rococo* perspectives. But we can nonetheless recognize the interest of the drawing as a record of someone's face by accepting that Watteau's drawing is—relative to the face-related portions of the drawing's content, anyway—a distinctively sensory record★ in relation to the *early rococo* perspectives. And we can express our reluctance to take Figure 4.5 to be a faithful reproduction of all of its subject's clothing by not accepting that—relative to, say, the left thigh-related portions of the picture's content—the drawing is a distinctively sensory record★ in relation to the *early rococo* perspectives. Similarly, while apparently recollective sensory mental images may not always impress themselves upon us as being distinctively sensory records in relation to domains of past perspectives, they at least present themselves as being distinctively sensory record★s.

To avoid tiresome occurrences of 'pretty much' and similar qualifying phrases, I have chosen to concentrate upon distinctively sensory records throughout most of this chapter. But the later discussions of distinctively sensory records could usually be rewritten so that they concerned distinctively sensory record★s instead of distinctively sensory records. The demanding nature of distinctively sensory recordhood therefore does not really limit the interest of the examinations of distinctively sensory records which follow. The distinction between distinctively sensory record★s and distinctively sensory records is important enough, however, that I have included some footnotes discussing its relevance to issues considered in the text. The next two sections return to the main issues of this chapter, by exploring some of the relationships between distinctively sensory records and causation.

---

[5] A bit more fully, suppose for example that P has the following form: *things stand sensorily way T from* _. Then our chosen distinctively sensory representation is a distinctively sensory record★ in relation to D, relative to P, just in case the following content is true relative to whatever standards of similarity happen to be in force: *there was a perspective x in D such that things stood sensorily from x some way that is suitably similar to T.*

Factoring out causation

There are important causal elements in many of the most obvious cases in which we seem to be put in touch with the past upon interacting with distinctively sensory records.

Playbacks of documentary film footage and daydreamed recollections of childhood days spent outside, for example, are alike in partly being products of the past events which they present to us. Those causal aspects of the previous examples are unsurprising, given that part of what is striking about them is the way in which they all apparently connect us to past events in a 'quasi-perceptual' manner. After all, a sensation counts as a perception—as a genuine seeing or hearing, say—only if the sensory episode has suitable causal connections to the world.

But the quasi-perceptual character of the instances currently of interest does not depend exclusively upon causal factors. Reconsider one of the images reproduced in the earlier chapters of this book: the drawing after Rembrandt reproduced as Figure 4.2, for instance. Suppose that you come to be convinced that, just as it happens, the ways that Figure 4.2 shows things as looking are ways that things in fact looked from some perspectives located in Sheffield during 1979. Imagine, that is, that you come to regard Figure 4.2 as being, by complete chance, a distinctively visual record in relation to the 1979-Sheffield perspectives.

Your beliefs about the drawing mean that, from your standpoint, there are some important respects in which its status is no different to that belonging to, say, what you believe to be a playback of documentary film footage. For it, too, captures how things once were in a particular part of the world, in an especially visual manner. But suppose too that your dealings with Figure 4.2 somehow lead you to *know* that the picture just happens to show what things once looked like from some 1979-Sheffield perspectives. Then there is a sense in which your comprehending views of the picture provide you with 'glimpses of the past' just as much as would, for instance, suitable views of documentary film footage.

For, by assumption, you know that the ways that the picture shows things as looking are ways that things once looked from some 1979-Sheffield perspectives. But *distinctively sensory showing comes from subjective informativeness.* Your grasp of the picture's distinctively visual content thus means that, in the course of your views of the picture, you appreciate what it is like to have sensations in which things look the ways that the picture shows things as looking. Your assumed knowledge of the ways that things once looked from some 1979-Sheffield perspectives, as mediated by your grasp of Figure 4.2's distinctively visual content, therefore has some important resemblances to your visually mediated knowledge of your current environment.[6]

On account of the very visual sensations which you are now having, for example, you know that things are currently *thus*. Similarly, as you look at the centre of Figure 4.2, your grasp of a portion of the picture's distinctively visual content means that you are thereby aware that the picture shows things as looking like *that*. You consequently know that, from some 1979-Sheffield perspective, things once looked like *that*.

Those points explain why causal considerations are to some extent irrelevant to the thought that suitable encounters with distinctively sensory records connect us to past events in a quasi-perceptual manner. And the explanation's overall shape—its insistence that the especially sensory nature of the contents of distinctively sensory records is partly what explains their special role in linking us to the past—seems right. So, to return to an earlier example, the emotional worth of family snapshots is not just owed to the causal relationships in which the photographs stand to past events: their importance also derives from the fact that the photos allow us to 'look back' into the past by *showing* us how things once looked.

As noted at the start of this section, however, causal matters do loom large when one considers a lot of the most striking examples of distinctively sensory records. What sorts of special roles do causal facts play in those cases? The following section identifies an important variety of causal chains that is implicated in the production of many striking types of distinctively sensory records.

A kind of causal chains

Listen for a moment to the things that are taking place around you. Next, use auditory mental images to recall what things were just like in your vicinity. The apparently recollective auditory mental images which you

---

[6] Similar remarks apply at this point to those distinctively sensory representations which are known to be distinctively sensory record★s but which are not distinctively sensory records; although in those cases the similarities to examples of sensorily mediated knowledge will be more attenuated, on account of the fact that the ways that the relevant representations show things as standing sensorily are merely suitably similar to ways that things once stood sensorily from relevant past perspectives.

just conjured were the product of a chain of causally linked factors, a chain which features the auditory sensations which you had a few moments ago but which does not start with them.

For let's suppose that those auditory sensations, in which things seemed to you to be certain ways, were auditory perceptions of things as being those ways. Then the ways that things sounded to you, in the course of the auditory sensations, were ways that things actually sounded from the perspectives at which your hearings occurred. Moreover, the causal conditions built into what it is for a sensation to be a genuine perception mean that the following holds: for each of the ways that things sounded to you in the course of your earlier auditory sensations, things sounded to you that way *because* things actually sounded that way from the perspective which you were occupying.

The ways that your earlier apparently recollective auditory mental images showed things as sounding were, I shall assume, faithful to your initial auditory sensations. That is, the ways that the images showed things as sounding were ways that things did sound to you in the course of your recent auditory sensations. Furthermore, the fact that the auditory mental images showed things as sounding those ways derived from the fact that things sounded those ways to you in the course of the earlier sensations.

There was therefore a short causal chain leading from the audible properties of the events in your recent environment to the auditory mental images which you produced some moments ago. And the character of the links in that chain ensured that the ways that the auditory mental images showed things as sounding were ways that things really did sound from the past perspectives in which your recent auditory sensations occurred. The nature of the links ensured, that is, that the auditory mental images were distinctively sensory records in relation to those past perspectives.

Causal chains of that general sort are very common. The ways that playbacks of documentary film footage show things as looking, for example, often are—and, moreover, are often causally dependent upon—ways that things actually looked from perspectives located at the places from where the footage was shot. As a result, those playbacks are distinctively sensory records in relation to domains including the perspectives located at the places and times where and when the footage was shot.[7] Similarly, the

---

[7] Relationships of counterfactual dependence are often cited in recent philosophical discussions of photography, particularly in the wake of Walton's provocative arguments for

ways that playbacks of audio recordings show things as sounding frequently are, and are causally dependent upon, ways that things actually sounded from perspectives situated at the places where the recordings were made.[8]

The causal chains just cited were especially simple in that, for each of the chains, the same ways for things to stand sensorily were passed along each of the links of the chain. But more complex causal chains of the same broad type are also possible.

A photo might be fed into a computer, for instance, to produce a distinctively visual representation whose content is a rule-governed transformation of the distinctively visual content of the original photo. And the relevant rules might guarantee the following: if the photo is a distinctively sensory record in relation to some domain of past perspectives, the representation resulting from the computerized process is also a distinctively sensory record in relation to some domain of past perspectives. The rules might ensure that, say, the ways that the distinctively sensory records produced by the process will show things as looking will be ways that things really did look from some perspectives simultaneous with, but about a yard to the right of, the perspectives from which things looked as the original photo shows them as looking.

Suppose that we are given a causal chain which leads to a distinctively sensory representation. And suppose that the ways that the resulting representation shows things as standing sensorily are causally dependent upon ways that things actually stood sensorily from certain past perspectives; where those causal dependencies ensure that the ways that the

---

the conclusion that 'we *see*, quite literally, our dead relatives themselves when we look at photographs of them' (Walton 1984, 86). The relationships thereby invoked tend to combine both ways in which the *visual appearances* of photographs themselves are dependent upon what things are like at the times at which the photographs are taken and ways in which the *contents* of photographs are dependent upon what things are like at the times at which the photographs are taken; see, for example, Walton 1984, 99–101, and Currie 1995, 53–6. By focusing exclusively upon content-based dependencies, however, we may track relationships of causal dependence which apply across a considerably broader range of cases—ones which apply to sensory mental images, for instance.

[8] Related sorts of causal chains may be implicated in the production of mere distinctively sensory record*s. Those chains can, however, allow for some slippage between the ways that the distinctively sensory record*s at the chains' ends show things as standing sensorily and the ways that things actually stood sensorily from the perspectives found in the circumstances standing at the start of the relevant chains. (Distinctively sensory record*s may also be produced by means of analogues of the more complex sorts of causal chains which are very soon to be discussed in the text.)

representation shows things as standing sensorily are ways that things actually once stood sensorily from some past perspectives. Then the causal chain is *sensorily preservative*. Next, assume that some process is capable of generating distinctively sensory records in the manner just sketched; that is, by producing distinctively sensory representations which stand at the end of sensorily preservative causal chains. Then I shall say that the process itself is *capable of being sensorily preservative*.

Epistemological dimensions

A wide range of familiar processes are capable of being sensorily preservative, and hence of linking us to the past in an especially intimate and direct way: traditional photographic methods, digital photographic techniques, sound recording processes, the production of handmade pictures using painting and drawing, the processes which yield our apparent sensory memories . . .

Our conceptions of what things were like in the past are often founded upon the outputs of processes that are capable of being sensorily preservative. Yet there are significant differences in the epistemological standings which we typically accord to the products of different processes that are alike in their capability of being sensorily preservative. This section and the next one will explore a couple of aspects of those differences. The aims of the sections are, in a sense, relatively modest: they are just intended, first, to illustrate how the framework articulated above may improve our understanding of various specific epistemic contrasts, by helping us to embed the latter within more general epistemological contexts; and, second, to suggest some promising lines of approach to the relevant epistemological contrasts.

Photographs are commonly taken to have an evidential value in relation to putative past facts which is not shared by drawings. (That said, the gap between photos and drawings seems clearly to have shrunk somewhat in the light of the development of digital photography.) It is tempting to think that the epistemic differences between photos and drawings partly reflect a contrast between the automatic nature of the former and the non-automatic nature of the latter. (Digital photography then muddies the waters because of the opportunities for human intervention which it makes available.)

Many processes are capable of producing pictures that look photo-graphic to us. But the evidential status of photographs does not just flow from what they look like. Paintings may look like photographs, for instance, but paintings have the same sort of evidential standing as drawings.[9] The special evidential standing of photographs is a product of the special epi-stemic standing of appropriate photographic processes. In particular, for those of us of a certain age the technologies by means of which traditional non-digital photographs are produced provide the paradigms that drive our faith in photographs as reliable documents of past times.

Traditional photography belongs to a broad class of processes that are capable of being sensorily preservative. In particular, photography using traditional cameras employs a process that proceeds automatically once it is set in motion, and along a series of well-understood physical pathways. There are numerous other processes that are capable of being sensorily preservative and which we know to fall into the same broad camp: there are methods of sound recording that belong there, for instance, and the same applies to suitably straightforward methods for producing digital photographs.

Suppose that we wish to establish how things stood sensorily from some past perspectives within a certain domain D. And assume that we are given a device whose proper functioning involves a process of the general 'automatic' sort roughed out in the previous paragraph. Suppose, finally, that the device was used to produce an item which, as we know, will have been a distinctively sensory record in relation to D so long as the device was working properly. Then the straightforward mechanics of the

---

[9] There are some interesting examples of photographic processes which people often interpret as producing distinctively sensory records, and which people treat as epistemically privileged for certain purposes, yet which are not generally sensorily preservative. Maynard 1997 examines photo-finish photography, for instance: the innocent viewer takes photo-finish photographs to show how things looked at a single moment; but in fact photo-finish photography usually employs photographic film moving past a narrow open slit to supply information about the state of a single part of space—the finish line—over an extended period. (The latter fact means that, when everything is working properly, the images resulting from the process may be trusted to reveal who crosses the finish line first, even though the image probably does not show how things actually looked from near to the finish line at the moment that the first person crossed the line.) The family of photographic processes thus encompasses a range of methods for producing photographs which differ from one another at fairly deep levels. In particular, the family of photographic processes that are intended to be sensorily preservative is, in some respects, fundamentally different from the family of photo-graphic processes that are meant to 'facilitate detection' (Maynard 1997) in other ways.

device mean that we may be able to gather good evidence that the automatic processes through which the machine produces distinctively sensory records would have proceeded smoothly at all of the times that are relevant to the perspectives in D. We may be able to test it to see whether it is now working properly, whether it has been altered recently, and so on.

By contrast, assume that some person has fashioned by hand a distinctively sensory representation. And suppose that the person claims that the representation is a distinctively sensory record in relation to D, on the basis of some sensations which she had during her occupation of perspectives drawn from D. The special roles of human agency in the distinctively sensory representation's genesis means that there are numerous characteristic points at which the causal chain leading to the representation may have failed to be sensorily preservative. And the peculiar nature of the possible failures generally makes it very hard to show decisively that they did not occur.[10]

The representation's maker might have intentionally ensured that the representation does not capture how things stood sensorily from any of the perspectives in D, for example; maybe she has a vested interest in the business. Alternatively, she might have failed without malice to capture any ways for things to stand sensorily which were suitably related to the ways that things stood sensorily for her; maybe she is bad at recalling what her sensations were like. Finally, the ways that things stood sensorily for the representation's producer might not have had anything to do with the ways that things actually stood sensorily from the perspectives in D; perhaps her sensory powers were totally deranged throughout the relevant period.[11]

Assume, then, that we are considering the question of what things were like around some past perspectives drawn from D. It is reasonable for us to be wary of relying upon somebody's claim to have produced by hand a

---

[10] The relative weakness of the conditions whose satisfaction are required for distinctively sensory record*hood means, in turn, that the conditions which need to be met if we are to show decisively that some handmade putative distinctively sensory record* is indeed a distinctively sensory record* are less stringent than the corresponding conditions for handmade putative distinctively sensory records; but the essentials of the following discussion nonetheless apply there too.

[11] See Abell 2010, 96, for some further discussion of the sorts of considerations currently being considered, in relation to the production of drawings in particular.

distinctively sensory record which captures what things were like around perspectives in D, particularly if the stakes are sufficiently high. But we may sensibly be less leery of accepting that the distinctively sensory representations owed to an automatic process of the sort illustrated by traditional photography are distinctively sensory records in relation to D. For we have a better chance, in that last case, of gathering good evidence that the causal chains eventually leading to the device's outputs were sensorily preservative.

The previous points may obviously be combined with salient differences between the processes through which photographs and drawings are produced, to explain some of the differences in the ways that we treat photographs and drawings as evidence for facts about the past.[12] The considerations outlined above also correctly predict that playbacks of suitable audio recordings would commonly be regarded as having more prima facie weight as evidence about the past than would, say, someone's attempt to use oral mimicry to capture what things sounded like from some past perspectives that he himself occupied.

Note, though, that the epistemic privileges belonging to the putative distinctively sensory records resulting from photography-like processes seem to depend upon the availability of relatively detailed information concerning the mechanics of the relevant processes. For the availability

---

[12]   Cohen and Meskin characterize the 'traditional explanation' for the epistemic standing of photography as being that 'photography is an inherently realistic medium' (2008, 70); it is not an explanation that they endorse. The approach to pictorial lifelikeness developed in Chapter 7 accounted for some important informational properties of lifelike pictures. The account explained, first, why the ways that lifelike pictures show things as looking tend to capture pretty significant ranges of those details which would seem to be seen by subjects to whom things really looked the ways that the pictures show things as looking. And the account explained, second, why one who grasps the distinctively visual content of a lifelike picture thereby gains a relatively rich appreciation of what it would really be like to have visual sensations in which things look the ways that the picture shows things as looking. Now suppose that some lifelike photograph—or any other lifelike picture, for that matter—is a distinctively sensory record in relation to a certain domain of past perspectives. Given the first of the above points about lifelikeness, it follows that the ways that the photo shows things as looking tend to provide bodies of distinctively visual information whose level of detail approximates significantly the level of detail present in the information which suitable views of a past scene would have disclosed to its viewers. And, given the second of the above points, it also follows that the photo has the power to give comprehending viewers of the photo a relatively rich sense of what it might really have been like to see a scene from the past. The ideas about lifelikeness developed earlier thus explain why the lifelikeness of lifelike photographs, and of lifelike pictorial distinctively sensory records more broadly, may contribute greatly to their value as sources of knowledge about the past.

of that information is what makes it feasible for us to gather sufficiently strong evidence that specific implementations of the processes incorporated sensorily preservative causal chains.[13]

Those last points may be linked to another epistemological contrast, a contrast that is philosophically more weighty than the one just considered. The processes which generate photographs, sound recordings, and related forms of distinctively sensory representations are just as automatically and reliably sensorily preservative as the processes which lead to our apparent sensory memories. And the detailed workings of the former processes are much better understood than the detailed workings of the latter process. It is consequently often easier to gather strong evidence indicating that photographs and the like are distinctively sensory records than it is to gather analogous evidence in relation to apparently recollective sensory mental images.

Yet it is natural to regard the processes which generate our apparent sensory memories as being a more basic source of justified beliefs concerning the past than, say, photography. In that respect, the apparently recollective sensory mental images figuring in apparent sensory memories seem to be more fully quasi-perceptual than photos, because it is also tempting to assume that perception is one of our basic sources of justified beliefs. What accounts for the special epistemic standing of apparent sensory memories as opposed to the products of—better understood and no less reliably sensorily preservative—processes like photography?

Further epistemological dimensions

Summon an apparent sensory memory of your childhood, one revolving around a visual mental image. The occurrence of the apparently recollective visual mental image involved its *seeming* to you that things were once a certain way, just as your current visual sensations involve its *seeming* to you that things are now a certain way. The visual mental image was thus the vehicle by means of which a certain existentially quantified past-directed content—one constructed upon a distinctively

---

[13] Cohen and Meskin argue that the special epistemic status that we accord to photographs, as opposed to say drawings, partly flows from our possession of relevant background beliefs about photographs as a type (2004, 205); they also cite the salience, in a certain sense, of photographs as a type for viewers of photographs within our culture.

visual content in the manner discussed earlier in this chapter—was presented to you as true.[14]

Compare the above case with what occurs when one idly views photographs. When you first viewed Figure 8.1, for example, you may have been inclined to form beliefs about the past. But your tendency to form those beliefs derived from your having learned that photographs often capture how things once looked, along with your recognition that Figure 8.1 is a photo. Our encounters with photographs do not involve past-directed appearances which are counterparts of the past-directed appearances generated by apparently recollective sensory mental images, or indeed of the present-directed appearances which figure in apparent perceptions.

Following Burge, let's say that 'entitlements are epistemic rights or warrants that need not be understood by or even accessible to the subject'.[15] Burge holds that we are entitled to rely upon perception,[16] for example. So, a young child may know next to nothing about how vision works, with the result that she lacks a lot of the resources—whatever they turn out to be!—which she would need to construct an explicit justification for the many beliefs which she bases directly upon what she seems to see. Yet, Burge claims, she nonetheless has an epistemic right to those beliefs; they are not poorly grounded.

Why might we be entitled to form beliefs on the basis of sensory episodes? The beliefs which we are entitled to form in the light of our sensations are presumably ones whose contents suitably reflect the ways that things look to us to be when we seem to see things. But if we are entitled to form those last beliefs, that is surely because we have a prior entitlement to trust that things are the ways that they look to us to be. Maybe, therefore, the primary entitlement which we have in relation to sensory episodes is an entitlement to trust any sensory appearances which the episodes involve.[17]

---

[14] The discussion in the text assumes that your apparently recollective visual mental image purported to show how things once stood sensorily from some past perspectives, rather than to show how things once stood sensorily in the course of some past sensations. There is further discussion below of the distinction between those apparently recollective sensory mental images that purport to show how things once stood from perspectives and those that purport to show how things once stood in the course of sensations.

[15] Burge 1993, 458.

[16] 'We are entitled to rely, other things being equal, on perception, memory, deductive and inductive reasoning, and on—I will claim—the word of others' (Burge 1993, 458).

[17] Pryor (2000, 547, footnote 37) seems to suggest something like the view that we are entitled to trust sensory appearances.

Suppose that to be true. Then the relevant entitlement might be basic; that is, it might not derive from any more general entitlement. On the other hand, however, the entitlement might flow from some more general entitlement of which it is a special instance.

Here is a more general entitlement from which it might flow. Sensory appearances are not the only sorts of appearances which we enjoy. Our apparent sensory memories involve appearances relating to how things once were, for example; and some have held that we enjoy more purely intellectual kinds of appearances. (Gödel, for instance, famously asserted that 'despite their remoteness from sense experience, we do have something like a perception of the objects of set theory, *as is seen from the fact that the axioms force themselves on us as being true*'.[18]) It might be held, then, that our entitlement to trust *sensory appearances* is merely an instance of our more general entitlement to trust *appearances*.

That proposal would obviously need refining. In particular, the 'appearances' to which it applies would need somehow to be circumscribed, so as to include only ones which are suitably analogous to sensory appearances. But let's suppose that the refinements can be made. And let's make the plausible assumption that the past-directed appearances figuring in apparent sensory memories would end up falling on the same side of the fence as sensory appearances.

The general entitlement to trust appearances would then imply, more specifically, that we are entitled to trust the past-directed appearances which feature in our apparent sensory memories. The general entitlement would imply, that is, that we are entitled to accept the existentially quantified past-directed contents which our apparently recollective sensory mental images serve to present to us as true. The general entitlement would not imply, however, that one is automatically entitled to regard photos like Figure 8.1 as being distinctively sensory records; and it is very hard to see what other remotely plausible principle of entitlement could have that last implication.

Are there any more general putative principles of entitlement worth considering at this point? Burge himself endorses an extremely general principle of entitlement, one that he calls the 'Acceptance Principle' and which runs thus: '*A person is entitled to accept as true something that is presented*

---

[18] Gödel 1964, 271; emphasis added.

as true and that is intelligible to him, unless there are stronger reasons not to do so.'[19]
The Acceptance Principle implies that we are entitled to trust sensory
appearances and the past-directed appearances incorporated within our
apparent sensory memories, for those are both varieties of episodes in
which intelligible contents are presented to us as true. And the Acceptance
Principle has further interesting implications.

I stated above that the ways that Figure 8.1 shows things as looking are
ways that things looked from some 2010-Northampton perspectives.
My assertion was an example of pictorially effected testimony. It is not
crazy to hold that you were entitled to regard the photo as being a
distinctively sensory record upon comprehending my assertion, even if
one is not generally just entitled to regard photos as being distinctively
sensory records. For it is not crazy to think that we are entitled to accept
instances of testimony, given that testimony is one of our most basic
sources of information about the world.

But the Acceptance Principle gives that result. For, as emphasized in
Chapter 2's initial discussions of sensory appearances, assertions are another
variety of episode in which contents are presented as true; and the content
which I presented as true when I made my earlier picture-citing assertion
was intelligible to you. While Burge's Acceptance Principle is justly
controversial, then, it may lead us to nuanced epistemological ideas relating to putative distinctively sensory records.[20]

Philosophical issues concerning the evidential status of, say, photographs, of drawings, and of apparent sensory memories feel like issues
that ought to be treated within broader contexts. But where exactly? By
treating the processes that generate photographs, drawings, and apparent
sensory memories as merely exemplifying categories of processes that are
capable of being sensorily preservative, we may isolate broader philosophical questions that are dramatized by, but not essentially bound to, representations of those more specific kinds. The earlier framework of ideas thus
helps us to embed our theoretical approaches to various relatively specific
phenomena within illuminating general contexts, by allowing us better to

---

[19] Burge 1993, 467; this is actually the 'first approximation' to the full Acceptance
Principle, which Burge enunciates on p. 469.

[20] So, numerous writers have objected to Burge's claim that we are entitled to trust
testimony: see, for example, Christensen and Kornblith 1997 (to which Burge 1997 responds)
and Faulkner 2000.

understand what many very different but nonetheless related sorts of processes hold in common.

There are various directions in which the ideas about distinctively sensory records developed above may be further generalized. The rest of the current chapter explores some of the additional extrapolations which can be made. It also illustrates some applications of the resulting ideas. The following section develops an unusually catholic position concerning the contents of apparent sensory memories.

Two types of apparent sensory memories

Sometimes, when one enjoys an apparent sensory memory, one seems to recall a sensory episode from one's own past. You can probably use auditory mental imagery to recall some way that things just sounded to you, for instance. But not all of our apparent sensory memories take that subjective form.

Consider your apparent sensory memories of things which happened at school during your adolescence. When you entertain those apparent sensory memories, it seems to you that certain events occurred during the course of your life. But can you honestly say that each of the apparent sensory memories involves its seeming to you that things once stood sensorily for you the very ways that the apparent sensory memory's accompanying sensory mental images show things as standing sensorily?[21] Does each of the apparently recollective visual mental images involved in the apparent sensory memories really seem to capture how things once looked *to you*?

Note, in this connection, that many apparent sensory memories are 'observer memories': apparent memories whose accompanying apparently recollective visual mental images display *oneself* as part of the apparently recalled scene.[22] But—just to take the cases that I know best—my own

---

[21] In the light of the earlier distinction between distinctively sensory record*s and distinctively sensory records, we should allow for memories whose featured sensory mental images seem merely to show us pretty much how things stood sensorily for us in the course of earlier sensory episodes. The common type of cases described in the next paragraph demonstrates that the apparently recollective sensory mental images figuring in our apparent sensory memories do not even always generate appearances of that broader subjective variety.

[22] For psychological discussion, see for example Nigro and Neisser 1983, Robinson and Swanson 1993, and McIsaac and Eich 2002; for interesting philosophical discussion, see

observer memories do not involve its seeming to me that things once looked to me the ways that the visual mental images show things as looking. Rather, they involve its seeming to me that there were once past scenes in which I played a certain part and which looked—'from somewhere' rather than 'to someone'—the ways that the visual mental images show things as looking.

Suppose that someone undergoes an apparent sensory memory which *does not* involve its seeming to the person that she once had sensations in which things stood sensorily the ways that some of the memory's accompanying sensory mental imagery shows things as standing sensorily. Then the apparent sensory memory is *external*. By contrast, suppose that someone undergoes an apparent sensory memory in which it *does* seem to the person that he once underwent sensations in which things stood sensorily the ways that some of the memory's accompanying sensory mental imagery shows things as standing sensorily. Then the apparent sensory memory is *internal*.

Sensation-characterizing distinctively sensory contents are no less gappy than perspective-characterizing ones. Existential quantifiers ranging over domains of past sensations may therefore be used to plug the gaps in sensation-characterizing distinctively sensory contents. The existentially quantified contents thereby produced are past-directed; but their import relates, more specifically, to how things once stood sensorily in the course of past sensory episodes. Those last points, along with some of the earlier ideas used in articulating the notion of a distinctively sensory record, make it easy to handle the distinction between external apparent sensory memories and internal apparent sensory memories.

Consider, first, an external apparent sensory memory. The memory's accompanying apparently recollective sensory mental images should be regarded as possessing exclusively perspective-characterizing distinctively sensory contents: that is, the relevant sensory mental images merely show things as standing sensorily certain ways from perspectives. The distinctively sensory contents belonging to the sensory mental images may serve as

Debus 2007 (although I am unsympathetic to the view which Debus develops to account for the possibility of observer memories, on which 'the spatial perspectival characteristics of' apparent sensory memories 'depend on the spatial perspectival characteristics of the perceptual experiences that the subject has at the time' when the apparent sensory remembering itself occurs (Debus 2007, 173)).

the bases for existentially quantified past-directed contents, as noted earlier in this chapter. The resulting contents relate to how things once stood sensorily from perspectives belonging to domains of past perspectives.

The past-directed appearances involved in external apparent sensory memories are then episodes in which particular past-directed contents of that type are presented to the subject as true, through the occurrence of apparently recollective sensory mental images within the subject's mind. But the contents thereby presented as true relate solely to how things once stood sensorily from domains of past perspectives. The sensory mental images accompanying external apparent sensory memories therefore *do not* serve ostensibly to portray how things once stood sensorily for the subjects of the apparent sensory memories.[23]

By contrast, internal apparent sensory memories feature apparently recollective sensory mental images which possess sensation-characterizing distinctively sensory contents. Their associated past-directed appearances are, again, episodes in which existentially quantified past-directed contents that are based upon the images' distinctively sensory contents are presented as true. But the existentially quantified past-directed contents thereby presented as true relate to how things once stood sensorily for someone. More precisely, the existential quantifiers involved in the past-directed contents range over domains of past sensory episodes enjoyed by the apparent sensory memory's subject. The sensory mental images featured in internal apparent sensory memories therefore *do* serve ostensibly to portray how things once stood sensorily for the subject of the apparent sensory memory.[24]

---

[23] The past-directed contents which are presented as true in the course of external apparent sensory memories may nonetheless feature some sort of reference to the subjects of the apparent memories; the crucial point is merely that external apparent sensory memories do not involve its seeming to the subject that things once stood sensorily for him or her *as the memory's apparently recollective sensory mental imagery shows things as standing sensorily*. So, for example, consider the existential quantifiers featuring in an existentially quantified past-directed content that is presented to someone as being true in the course of an external apparent sensory memory. I think that it is very plausible that the domains of perspectives over which those existential quantifiers range are, within the existentially quantified past-directed content, characterized in relation to the very subject of the apparent sensory memory. (Burge 2003 argues forcefully that the contents of all sensory memories have *de se* elements.)

[24] The range of cases just identified in the text involve analogues of putative distinctively sensory records; but the category of instances is easily widened to encompass sensation-characterizing counterparts of distinctively sensory record*s.

Or just one?

Despite the fact that it seems introspectively clear that there may be both internal and external apparent sensory memories, philosophical discussions of apparent sensory memories have commonly evinced a presumption that apparent sensory memories must either always be internal or always be external.[25]

Husserl moves from one extreme to the other, for example. He writes at one time that '[t]he following is an evident proposition: Every memory of an A is at the same time the memory of an earlier perception of the A'.[26] Yet he comments at a later date that '[m]emory does actually imply a reproduction of the earlier perception, but the memory is not in the proper sense a representation of it: the perception is not meant and posited in the memory; what is meant and posited is the perception's object and the object's now, which, in addition, is posited in relation to the actually present now'.[27]

And Broad, after outlining something like the view that apparent sensory memories are always internal, puts alongside it something like the hypothesis that they are always external, eventually stating that he does 'not feel able to make up [his] mind on the question'[28] which of the approaches is correct—having thus ignored the possibility that some apparent sensory memories are internal but some are external.

The 'exclusivist' tendency is most commonly embodied, however, in the more specific belief that apparent sensory memories must always be internal. Locke, for instance, asserts that memory is the mind's capacity 'to revive Perceptions, which it has once had, with this additional perception

---

[25] In thinking about the contents of the past-directed appearances which accompany apparent sensory memories, it is natural to move outwards from the contents of their constituent apparently recollective sensory mental images, as I have done. But, as we have seen in earlier chapters, one might wonder how it is possible for some sensory mental images to portray sensations and for others not to portray sensations. If one cannot see any way of sensibly allowing for both of those possibilities, one may consequently assume that apparent sensory memories must either always be internal or always be external. The presumption noted in the text is therefore a fairly natural one if one does not have to hand something like the distinction between perspective-characterizing and sensation-characterizing distinctively sensory contents.

[26] Husserl [1898–1925] 2005, 236, writing around 1898.

[27] Husserl [1893–1917], 1990, 60, writing in 1905.

[28] Broad 1929, 240–1.

annexed to them, that it has had them before'.[29] Owens construes Locke as stating that 'something experienced as a memory presents itself as an experience one has previously enjoyed',[30] a proposal which Owens himself endorses. Martin claims, meanwhile, that 'memory . . . [is] the representational recall of [a past] experiential encounter'.[31]

One recurrent strand in the reasoning which has led philosophers to the view that apparent sensory memories must always be internal is the thought that there cannot otherwise be a satisfactory account of the ways in which apparent sensory memories differ from distinct but related phenomena.

Owens, for example, argues that his view enables us to understand the difference between sensory episodes proper and apparent sensory memories, and also to understand the difference between mere recognition and apparent sensory recollection.[32] And Martin constructs a complicated argument for his position, which hinges upon the rejection of an assumption which will, he claims, lead its advocates 'to insist that any distinction in kind between [apparent sensory] recall and perceptual experience would have to be drawn in terms of something extrinsic to the experiential character of the episodes'.[33] It is therefore worth noting that we may, while treating external apparent sensory memories in the way proposed in the previous section, nonetheless hold external apparent sensory memories well apart from the related phenomena cited by Owens and Martin.

Sensory episodes and mere recognizings, for example, do not involve its seeming to us that things once stood sensorily certain ways from some past perspectives. There is therefore no danger of their being confused with external apparent sensory memories. Indeed, the specifically past-directed nature of the appearances involved in external apparent sensory memories means that the purported relationships which the latter have to the past are

---

[29] Locke [1690] 1975, 150.

[30] Owens 1996, 323. Owens's Lockean view seems to me to conflate the apparently recollective sensory mental images which figure in apparent sensory memories with aspects of the distinctively sensory contents of those images. For, while the relevant sensory mental images serve to present *the ways for things to stand sensorily* figuring in their distinctively sensory contents as (pretty much) ways that things once stood sensorily, it seems wrong to state that the sensory mental images are *themselves* presented to one as being past experiences which one enjoyed.

[31] Martin 2001, 270.

[32] See Owens 1996, 325–9.

[33] Martin 2001, 270; see pp. 269–79 of Martin's paper for the argument.

written into their very phenomenologies. The previous section's account of external apparent sensory memories thus allows us to distinguish between external apparent sensory memories and sensory episodes without supposing that, to requote Martin, the distinction between those cases must be drawn 'in terms of something extrinsic to the experiential character of the episodes' themselves.

Yet we may still recognize a kinship between external apparent sensory memories and genuine sensations. For, as discussed earlier in this chapter, the distinctively sensory nature of the contents which form the bases for the past-directed appearances involved in external apparent sensory memories means that external apparent sensory memories have a pronouncedly quasi-perceptual character.

Introspection strongly supports the view that there are both internal and external apparent sensory memories.[34] It must be confessed, however, that the idea that every apparent sensory memory is internal is less initially incredible than, say, the view that every picture must represent a visual sensation from the inside. But that is probably merely because our concept of memory demands that the sensorily preservative causal chains which lead to our genuine sensory memories should have at their inceptions sensory episodes in which we ourselves witnessed suitable things: one cannot have genuine sensory memories of happenings which one did not oneself witness.[35]

Recall that, when introducing the notion of a sensorily preservative causal chain, I distinguished the most straightforward range of cases—those in which ways for things to stand sensorily are passed unchanged along the links of the chain—from cases of a more complex transformative kind.

[34] As an aside, I think that introspection also supports the view that there are apparent sensory memories which are neither definitely internal nor definitely external. Those cases may be handled by treating the sensory mental images at their hearts as suffering from a radical form of representational indeterminacy. For they may be viewed as instances in which it is indeterminate whether the relevant sensory mental images show things as standing sensorily certain ways from perspectives or whether they show things as standing sensorily certain ways in the course of sensations.

[35] Having sniped at Broad for being an exclusivist, I should note that the indecision which manifests his exclusivism is in many ways laudable. He remarks that '[s]ince we all believe strongly that nothing can be remembered unless it has been perceived by us, we shall almost inevitably infer when we remember an event that we must have perceived it. And we may very well confuse this natural and immediate inference with a genuine memory-belief; and thus think that the proposition: "I have perceived this" was part of the content of the original memory-belief, when really it is a reflective and inferential addition' (Broad 1929, 240).

The latter range of instances was illustrated using the example of a photograph which, upon being fed into a computer, led to the production of a distinctively sensory record whose distinctively sensory content resulted from a rule-governed transformation of the distinctively sensory content belonging to the original photo.

The possibility of sensorily preservative causal chains of that second type is relevant to one of the major categories of external apparent sensory memories cited previously, namely observer memories. Observer memories come to us from sensations in which things stood sensorily certain ways for us. But the ways that things stood sensorily for us in the course of the relevant sensations evidently are not passed unchanged along the links of the chains that lead eventually to observer memories. Those ways for things to stand sensorily are, rather, transformed along the chain's length into ways that things stood sensorily from perspectives which were *nearby* to the ones which we ourselves occupied during the recalled episodes.[36]

The part played by transformative sensorily preservative causal chains in the production of observer memories illustrates how the ways that things are shown as having once stood sensorily by apparently recollective sensory mental images may derive from, yet leave behind, ways that things actually stood sensorily for us at earlier times. But we do not, in the cases resulting from transformative chains, inevitably suffer from illusions about what things were once like for us. For the past-directed appearances accompanying the resulting apparent sensory memories do not always purport to present us with characterizations of our earlier sensations; they often purport simply to tell us about the world as it was in the course of our lives.

Other directions

The account of distinctively sensory records which underpinned the earlier parts of this chapter depended upon various fundamental ideas. In particular, it started from the thought that distinctively sensory contents may, because of their gappy nature, form the bases of more complex contents. And it assumed that those more complex contents may feature

---

[36] Note that the above sentence is easily revised, using a well-placed 'pretty much', to cater for those observer memories whose apparently recollective sensory mental images are putative distinctively sensory record*s rather than putative distinctively sensory records.

in episodes in which the contents are presented with various kinds of force. The generality of those fundamental ideas means that they enable us to regard some of the phenomena examined above as being continuous with other intuitively related sorts of actual and possible phenomena. I shall close this chapter with some brief illustrations of that point.

Our apparent sensory memories are aimed towards the past. But there could be related mental capacities whose outputs pointed elsewhere. The idea of 'seeing into the future' by means of forward-looking counterparts of apparent sensory memories is not very exotic, for instance. It is a straightforward matter to adapt this chapter's treatment of apparent sensory memories to handle possible cases of that last kind. For the distinctively sensory contents of sensory mental images may be combined with existential quantifiers ranging over domains of future perspectives and sensations, to yield more complex future-directed contents. We may then regard the envisaged prophetic episodes as involving appearances in which such existentially quantified future-directed contents are presented to their subjects as being true.[37]

A final example: as noted in Chapter 6, Walton has sought to use the idea of make-believe in making sense of a plethora of important phenomena. I argued there that Walton's pretence-based approach to depiction does not provide a promising basis for an analysis of what it is to be a picture which shows things as looking certain ways. But the notion of make-believe might otherwise be useful in helping us to understand the representational roles sometimes played by distinctively sensory representations.

Consider, for instance, the illustrations which Leech provided for Surtees's classic nineteenth-century comic hunting novel, *Mr. Sponge's Sporting*

---

[37] One interesting possibility is that, when we produce sensory mental images with exclusively perspective-characterizing distinctively sensory contents, it may sometimes thereby appear to us that there *could be* perspectives from which things stood sensorily the ways that the sensory mental images show things as standing sensorily. If that is right (and it seems quite plausible to me), there is a restricted sense in which episodes featuring sensory mental imagery may provide us with 'appearances of possibility' whose contents relate to the external world. (The view that imaginings *always* involve 'appearances of possibility' is endorsed in Yablo 1993. Gregory 2010a rejects that thesis, on the basis of various sorts of cases which I still think refute it; that paper was written some time before I had worked out the ideas articulated in this book, however, and aspects of the paper's handling of the imagination could be improved.) Note too that, given the Burgean thesis that we are entitled to accept intelligible contents which are presented to us as true, one's ability to produce sensory mental images would then amount to a powerful source of well-grounded modal beliefs concerning how the outside world could be.

Tour.[38] Those pictures are not putative presentations of real scenes: Leech did not take the picture of 'Mr Jogglebury Crowdey with his dog and his gun'[39] to show how things look, have ever looked, or will look from any real perspectives. Yet if we are to do justice to the representational function of Leech's pictures, it does not seem to be sufficient merely to ascribe distinctively visual contents to them. For there is a sense in which the function of the pictures, in relation to the narrative, is too singular for that. Although the picture of Mr Jogglebury Crowdey in the field does not show how he looked, looks, or will look from any specific actual perspectives, it does show us how he looks from some specific fictional ones. But what is a 'specific fictional perspective'?

Make-believe may help us here. It does not seem unnatural to regard our attitude towards Leech's illustrations as leavened by a pinch of pretence. In reading the book—which is, like lots of novels, written in the past tense—and in looking at the accompanying pictures, perhaps we pretend that the images are distinctively sensory records in relation to a range of past perspectives that are suitably connected to some real past events which we pretend the novel to be recounting. In the case of illustrated stories set in the future, by contrast, perhaps we pretend that the illustrative images show how things will look from some future perspectives that are appropriately related to some real future events which we pretend the story to be describing. Related ideas may be applied to make sense of the representational functions of images in many narrative films, to take just one of lots of further relevant cases.

---

[38] Surtees [1854] 1981.   [39] Surtees [1854] 1981, between 330 and 331.

Conclusion

The bulk of this book's earlier parts aimed to show how ideas about distinctively sensory content may clarify and resolve a wide range of issues relating to distinctively sensory representations. The previous chapter broadened the book's perspective somewhat, however, by embedding its handling of distinctively sensory representations within a broader context, initially provided by reflection upon some of our standard sources of knowledge about the past. This brief conclusion will continue that trend, by sketching the wider philosophical relevance of some of the theorizing contained in Chapters 1–3.

The theory of distinctively sensory content developed previously deployed an array of background assumptions relating to types of sensations, sensory appearances, and perspectives. Some of the ideas thereby summoned were fairly familiar but some of them were more novel; and their more novel elements—in particular, the idea of a way that things stand sensorily from a perspective, as explicated in Chapter 2—may be used to generate new approaches towards aspects of our sensory experiences themselves.[1]

Husserl writes that:

[w]hen we view [a] table, we view it from some particular side, and this side is thereby what is genuinely seen. Yet the table has still other sides . . . [And] this thing is not [merely] the side genuinely seen in this moment; rather (according to the very sense of perception) the thing is precisely the full-thing that has still other sides, sides that are not brought to genuine perception in this perception, but that would be brought to genuine perception in other perceptions.[2]

---

[1] The example which follows is relevant to Chapter 2's assumption, in replying to the No Lookerless Looks argument, that the contents of visual appearances are commonly silent about mental matters.

[2] Husserl 2001, 40.

Husserl's remarks capture an important aspect of visual experience: our apparent seeings of external objects are typically intimately related to accompanying expectations concerning the ways that the apparently seen items would look to us if we were to shift our positions.

How best to cater for those connections? One might regard the expectations as mere accompaniments of the visual sensations, accompaniments which are not grounded in the intrinsic character of the visual sensations themselves. My current visual sensations are accompanied by expectations relating to what I am going to have for lunch, for example, although the presence of those last expectations tells us very little about vision. While that view might be correct, Husserl's comments suggest a stronger but still fairly appealing conception of the status of the expectations to which he refers. The expectations might be held somehow to mirror materials that are implicit within the visual sensations which the expectations accompany.

Husserl's talk about 'the very sense of perception' indicates a bullish way in which one might try to fill out that last thought: one might build the contents of the noted expectations into the contents of the visual appearances which they accompany. On this view, the contents of visual appearances usually include counterfactuals concerning the visual sensations which we would have under currently unrealized conditions. That position has recently been endorsed—it is advocated by Noë and Siegel, for example[3]—but it is somewhat implausible. Is there a way of yoking the expectations cited by Husserl to material that might more naturally be regarded as internal to the visual sensations with which the expectations are associated?

Look at the pages in front of you. You would be startled if, upon altering your position, the new ways that those pages then looked to you to be did not meet various conditions; you take it that they will not then look to be circular, for instance.

You appreciate, after all, that *if* the way that those pages now look to you is indeed a way that the pages look from your current perspective *then* the distinct ways that the pages look from other perspectives, simultaneous with and near to your own, meet various consequent conditions. But you also presume that the ways which the pages would look to you, if you

---

[3] See Noë 2004; and Siegel 2006.

were to occupy immediate descendants of the latter perspectives, would be ways that the pages actually now look from the relevant perspectives. For you presume that the properties of the pages will remain relatively constant in the immediate future; and you expect that your visual system will continue to work well during that period.

More generally, we might seek to accommodate the phenomena remarked by Husserl by holding that our expectations concerning the ways that things would look to us, if we were to move, are generally shaped by the following: first, our awareness of the implications which the ways that things look from *one* perspective sometimes have for the different ways that things look from *other* perspectives; and, second, our reliance upon background assumptions which connect the ways that things in fact look from certain *perspectives* to the ways that things would look *to us* if we were to change our positions in appropriate ways.

On the proposed approach, the noted expectations therefore do indeed reflect matter that is implicit within the visual sensations which they accompany. Yet the expectations do not derive from references within the contents of visual appearances to non-occurrent visual sensations. They flow instead from our ability to appreciate that a special kind of implicational relationship sometimes holds among ways for things to look. Needless to say, the mooted approach to Husserl's phenomena relies upon Chapter 2's distinction between the notion of a way that things look in the course of a visual sensation and the notion of a way that things look from a perspective.

The concept of distinctively sensory content proper also promises to have additional applications, some of which are more grand than those examined in previous chapters. In particular, to return to a theme first sounded in Chapter 1, while distinctively sensory contents were originally introduced by means of their relationships to distinctively sensory representations, the later theory of their special nature effectively provided an account of certain materials which commonly form part of the substance of thought and reasoning.

Many people have felt the need for cognitive intermediaries between occurrent sensations and relatively abstract forms of thought. The 'ideas' of the classical empiricists—the 'faint images' of 'impressions' in 'thinking and reasoning', in Hume's words[4]—were meant to provide a way in which the

---

[4] Hume [1739–40] 1978, 1.

stuff of occurrent sensations could be taken up in later thought, as were the 'schemata' posited by Kant.[5] More recently, 'neo-empiricist' psychologists have sought to show that 'cognition is inherently perceptual, sharing systems with perception at both the cognitive and neural levels';[6] and McDowell has claimed that, to make sense of the ways in which experience is evidentially relevant to rational thought, we need to accept that some of the conceptual matter of the latter is already found within the former.[7]

Numerous different pressures led those writers to their positions, and it would be quixotic to claim that the mere recognition of distinctively sensory contents could allay all of their concerns. But it is worth noting that distinctively sensory contents, regarded simply as aspects of information, look set to play an absolutely crucial role in our minds' lives, precisely on account of their potential to mediate between occurrent sensations and subsequent thought.

Distinctively sensory contents have, on the one hand, the power to preserve characteristically sensory aspects of sensory episodes. The fact that *distinctively sensory showing comes from subjective informativeness* means that subjective facets of sensations may live on in distinctively sensory representations, for instance; while the fact that *scene-showing corresponds to seeming* means that facts about what distinctively sensory representations show mirror the ways in which perceptions may present the outside world to us. On the other hand, distinctively sensory contents are able to abstract from specific sensations, because they incorporate more or less general ways for things to stand sensorily. Distinctively sensory contents are thus able to broker a compromise between the bustle of our sensory lives and the calmer abstractions of rational thought.

Those last points are impressionistic and they hardly amount to a compelling demonstration of the general importance of distinctively sensory contents as conciliators between sensory episodes and abstract varieties of thought. Yet it is surely independently plausible that we might, by summoning ideas about distinctively sensory content, broaden our underlying conceptions of the forms which aspects of information may

---

[5] Kant [1781 and 1787] 1999, 271–7; see Gardner 1999, 166–71, for helpful discussion.
[6] Barsalou 1999, 577.
[7] See, for example, Lecture 1 of McDowell 1994.

take, and hence enrich our conceptions of the shapes which cognition may assume. For, to return again to one of the themes announced in Chapter 1, the aspects of information which answer to the contents of distinctively sensory representations have been notably neglected by philosophers and others, despite their centrality to our understandings of the world and of ourselves.

References

Abell, C. (2007), 'Pictorial realism', *Australasian Journal of Philosophy* 85: 1–17.

Abell, C. (2009), 'Canny resemblance', *Philosophical Review* 183: 183–223.

Abell, C. (2010), 'The epistemic value of photographs', in Abell and Bantinaki (2010).

Abell, C. and K. Bantinaki (eds.) (2010), *Philosophical Perspectives on Depiction*, Oxford University Press: Oxford.

Alberti, L. B. ([1435–6] 1966), *On Painting*, trans. J. R. Spencer, Yale University Press: New Haven, CT.

Armstrong, D. M. (1962), *Bodily Sensations*, Routledge and Kegan Paul: London.

Arnheim, R. (1974), *Art and Visual Perception: A Psychology of the Creative Eye (The New Version)*, University of California Press: Berkeley, California.

Bahn, P. G. (1998), *The Cambridge Illustrated History of Prehistoric Art*, Cambridge University Press: Cambridge.

Barsalou, L. W. (1999), 'Perceptual symbol systems', *Behavioural and Brain Sciences* 22: 577–609.

Beaney, M. (ed.) (1997), *The Frege Reader*, Blackwell: Oxford.

Benacerraf, P. and H. Putnam (eds.) (1964), *Philosophy of Mathematics: Selected Readings*, Cambridge University Press: Cambridge.

Bermúdez, J. L. (1995), 'Nonconceptual content: from perceptual experience to subpersonal computational states', *Mind and Language* 10: 333–69.

Block, N. (ed.) (1981), *Imagery*, MIT Press: Cambridge, MA.

Blumson, B. (2010), 'Pictures, perspective and possibility', *Philosophical Studies* 149: 135–51.

Bois, Y.-A. (1992), 'The semiology of cubism', in Zelevansky (1992).

Brewer, B. (2006), 'Perception and content', *European Journal of Philosophy* 15: 165–81.

Broad, C. D. (1929), *The Mind and its Place in Nature*, Kegan Paul, Trench, Trubner, and Co. Ltd: London.

Budd, M. (1993), 'How pictures look', in Knowles and Skorupski (1993).

Bunzeck, N., T. Wuestenberg, K. Lutz, H. J. Heinze, and L. Jancke (2005), 'Scanning silence: mental imagery of complex sounds', *Neuroimage* 26: 1119–27.

Burge, T. (1993), 'Content preservation', *Philosophical Review* 102: 457–88.

Burge, T. (1997), 'Interlocution, perception, and memory', *Philosophical Studies* 86: 21–47.

Burge, T. (2003), 'Memory and persons', *Philosophical Review* 112: 289–337.

Burge, T. (2010), *Origins of Objectivity*, Oxford University Press: Oxford.

Casati, R. (2010), 'Hallucinatory pictures', *Acta Analytica* 25: 365–8.

Christensen, D. and H. Kornblith (1997), 'Testimony, memory and the limits of the a priori', *Philosophical Studies* 86: 1–20.

Clark, A. (2001), 'Visual experience and motor action: are the bonds too tight?', *Philosophical Review* 110: 495–519.

Clark, T. J. (1999), *Farewell to an Idea: Episodes from a History of Modernism*, Yale University Press: New Haven and London.

Cohen, J. and A. Meskin (2004), 'On the epistemic status of photographs', *Journal of Aesthetics and Art Criticism* 67: 197–210.

Cohen, J. and A. Meskin (2008), 'Photographs as evidence', in Walden (2008).

Conee, E. (1994), 'Phenomenal knowledge', *Australasian Journal of Philosophy* 72: 136–50.

Cowey, A. and E. T. Rolls (1974), 'Human cortical magnification factor and its relation to visual acuity', *Experimental Brain Research* 21: 447–54.

Crane, T. (1988), 'The Waterfall Illusion', *Analysis* 48: 142–7.

Currie, G. (1995), *Image and Mind: Film, Philosophy, and Cognitive Science*, Cambridge University Press: Cambridge.

Damasio, H., T. J. Grabowski, A. Damasio, D. Tranel, L. Boles-Ponto, G. L. Watkins, and R. D. Hickwa (1993), 'Visual recall with eyes closed and covered activates early visual cortex', *Neuroscience Abstracts* 19: 1603.

Debus, D. (2007), 'Perspectives on the past: a study of the spatial perspectival characteristics of recollective memories', *Mind and Language* 22: 173–206.

Denis, M. and S. M. Kosslyn (1999), 'Scanning visual images: a window on the mind', *Cahiers de Psychologie Cognitive/Current Psychology of Cognition* 18: 409–65.

Denis, M., E. Mellet, and S. M. Kosslyn (eds.) (2004), *Neuroimaging of Mental Imagery: A Special Issue of The European Journal of Cognitive Psychology*, Psychology Press: Hove.

Dretske, F. (1981), *Knowledge and the Flow of Information*, MIT Press: Cambridge, MA.

Duncan, R. O. and G. M. Boynton (2003), 'Cortical magnification within human primary visual cortex correlates with acuity thresholds', *Neuron* 38: 659–71.

Dupoux, E., S. Dehane, and L. Cohen (eds.) (2002), *Cognition: A Critical Look: Advances, Questions and Controversies in Honor of J. Mehler*, MIT Press: Cambridge, MA.

Evans, G. (1982), *The Varieties of Reference*, ed. J. McDowell, Clarendon Press: Oxford.

Faulkner, P. (2000), 'The social character of testimonial knowledge', *Journal of Philosophy* 97: 581–601.

Finke, R. A. (1989), *Principles of Mental Imagery*, MIT Press: Cambridge, MA.

Finke, R. A. and S. M. Kosslyn (1980), 'Mental imagery acuity in the peripheral visual field', *Journal of Experimental Psychology: Human Perception and Performance* 6: 244–64.

Foster, H., R. Krauss, Y.-A. Bois, and B. H. D. Buchloh (2004), *Art Since 1900*, Thames and Hudson Ltd: London.

Foster J. and H. Robinson (eds.) (1985), *Essays on Berkeley*, Clarendon Press: Oxford.

Frege, G. ([1891] 1997), 'Function and concept', in Beaney (1997).

Frege, G. ([1892a] 1997), 'On *Sinn* and *Bedeutung*', in Beaney (1997).

Frege, G. ([1892b] 1997), 'On concept and object', in Beaney (1997).

Frege, G. ([1904] 1980), 'What is a function?', in Geach and Black (1980).

Fry, E. F. (ed.) (1966), *Cubism*, Thames and Hudson Ltd: London.

Gardner, S. (1999), *Kant and the Critique of Pure Reason*, Routledge: London.

Geach, P. and M. Black (eds. and trans.) (1980), *Translations from the Philosophical Writings of Gottlob Frege*, Basil Blackwell: Oxford.

Gluck, M. A., J. R. Anderson, and S. M. Kosslyn (eds.) (2008), *Memory and Mind: A festschrift for Gordon H. Bower*, Erlbaum Associates: Hillsdale, NJ.

Gödel, K. (1964), 'What is Cantor's continuum problem?', in Benacerraf and Putnam (1964).

Goodman, N. (1969), *Languages of Art*, Oxford University Press: London.

Gregory, D. (2006), 'Functionalism about possible worlds', *Australasian Journal of Philosophy* 84: 95–115.

Gregory, D. (2010a), 'Conceivability and apparent possibility', in Hale and Hoffman (2010).

Gregory, D. (2010b), 'Pictures, pictorial contents and vision', *British Journal of Aesthetics* 50: 15–32.

Gregory, D. (2010c), 'Visual imagery: visual format or visual content?', *Mind and Language* 25: 394–417.

Gregory, D. (2010d), 'Imagery, the imagination and experience', *Philosophical Quarterly* 60: 735–53.

Gunther, Y. H. (ed.) (2003), *Essays on Nonconceptual Content*, MIT Press: Cambridge, MA.

Hale, B. and A. Hoffman (eds.) (2010), *Modality: Metaphysics, Logic, and Epistemology*, Oxford University Press: Oxford.

Handy, T. C., M. B. Miller, B. Schott, N. M. Shroff, P. Janata, J. D. Van Horn, S. Inati, S. T. Grafton, and M. S. Gazzaniga (2004), 'Visual imagery and memory: do retrieval strategies affect what the mind's eye sees?', in Denis, Mellet, and Kosslyn (2004).

Harman, G. (1990), 'The intrinsic quality of experience', *Philosophical Perspectives* 4: 31–52.

Haugeland, J. (1998), *Having Thought*, Harvard University Press: Cambridge, MA.

Hecht, H., R. Schwartz, and M. Atherton (eds.) (2003), *Looking into Pictures*, MIT Press: Cambridge, MA.

Heck, R. G. (2000), 'Nonconceptual content and the "space of reasons"', *Philosophical Review* 109: 483–523.

Heck, R. G. (2007), 'Are there different kinds of content?', in McLaughlin and Cohen (2007).

Hockney, D. (2006), *Secret Knowledge: Rediscovering the Lost Techniques of the Old Masters* (new and expanded edition), Thames and Hudson: London.

Hoerl, C. and T. McCormack (eds.) (2001), *Time and Memory*, Clarendon Press: Oxford.

Hopkins, R. (1995), 'Explaining depiction', *Philosophical Review* 104: 425–55.

Hopkins, R. (1998), *Picture, Image and Experience*, Cambridge University Press: Cambridge.

Hopkins, R. (2000), 'Touching pictures', *British Journal of Aesthetics* 40: 149–67.

Hume, D. ([1739–49] 1978), *A Treatise of Human Nature*, ed. L. A. Selby-Bigge and P. H. Nidditch (2nd edition), Clarendon Press: Oxford.

Husserl, E. ([1893–1917] 1990), *On the Phenomenology of the Consciousness of Internal Time (1893–1917)*, trans. J. B. Brough, Springer: Dordrecht.

Husserl, E. ([1898–1925] 2005), *Phantasy, Image Consciousness, and Memory (1898–1925)*, trans. J. B. Brough, Springer: Dordrecht.

Husserl, E. (2001), *Analyses Concerning Passive and Active Synthesis: Lectures on Transcendental Logic*, trans. A. J. Steinbock, Kulwer Academic Publishers: Dordrecht.

Hyman, J. (2006), *The Objective Eye: Color, Form and Reality in the Theory of Art*, University of Chicago Press: Chicago.

Hyman, J. (forthcoming), 'Depiction', to appear in a Royal Institute of Philosophy Supplement on *Philosophy and the Arts*.

Kant, I. ([1781 and 1787] 1999), *Critique of Pure Reason*, trans. and ed. P. Guyer and A. W. Wood, Cambridge University Press: Cambridge.

Karmel, P. (2003), *Picasso and the Invention of Cubism*, Yale University Press: New Haven and London.

Keefe, R. (2000), *Theories of Vagueness*, Cambridge University Press: Cambridge.

Klee, P. (1961), *The Thinking Eye: The Notebooks of Paul Klee*, vol. 1, ed. J. Spiller, trans. R. Mannheim, George Wittenborn: London.

Knowles, D. and J. Skorupski (eds.) (1993), *Virtues and Taste: Essays on Politics, Ethics and Aesthetics*, Basil Blackwell: Oxford.

Koerner, J. L. (2009), *Caspar David Friedrich and the Subject of Landscape* (2nd edition), Reaktion Books: London.

Kosslyn, S. M. (1973), 'Scanning visual images: some structural implications', *Perception and Psychophysics* 14: 90–4.

Kosslyn, S. M. (1980), *Image and Mind*, Harvard University Press: Cambridge, MA.

Kosslyn. S. M. (1981), 'The medium and the message in mental imagery', in Block (1981).

Kosslyn, S. M. (2008), 'Remembering images', in Gluck, Anderson, and Kosslyn (2008).

Kosslyn, S. M., T. M. Ball, and B. J. Reiser (1978), 'Visual images preserve metric spatial information: evidence from studies of image scanning', *Journal of Experimental Psychology: Human Perception and Performance* 4: 47–60.

Kosslyn, S. M., S. Pinker, G. E. Smith, and S. P. Shwartz (1979), 'On the demystification of mental imagery', *Behavioural and Brain Sciences* 2: 535–48; partially reprinted in Block (1981), to which all page references refer.

Kosslyn, S. M. and W. L. Thompson (2003), 'When is early visual cortex activated during visual mental imagery?', *Psychological Bulletin* 129: 723–46.

Kraemer, D. J. M., C. N. Macrae, A. E. Green, and W. M. Kelley (2005), 'Sound of silence activates auditory cortex', *Nature* 434: 158.

Krauss, R. (1992), 'The motivation of the sign', in Zelevansky (1992).

Kripke, S. (1981), *Naming and Necessity*, Basil Blackwell: Oxford.

Kulvicki, J. (2006), *On Images: Their Structure and Content*, Oxford University Press: Oxford.

Kulvicki, J. (2010), 'Pictorial diversity', in Abell and Bantinaki (2010).

Lamarque, P. and S. Haugom Olsen (eds.) (2004), *Aesthetics and the Philosophy of Art: The Analytic Tradition*, Blackwell Publishing: Oxford.

Le Bihan, D., R. Turner, T. A. Zeffiro, C. Cuénod, P. Jezzard, and V. Bonnerot (1993), 'Activation of human primary visual cortex during visual recall: a magnetic resonance imaging study', *Proceedings of the National Academy of Sciences U.S.A.* 90: 11802–5.

Lessing, G. E. ([1766] 2005), *Laocoön: An Essay upon the Limits of Painting and Poetry*, trans. E. Frothingham, Dover Publications: Mineola, NY.

Levinson, J. (1998) 'Wollheim on pictorial representation', *The Journal of Aesthetics and Art Criticism* 56: 227–33.

Lewis, D. K. (1973), *Counterfactuals*, Basil Blackwell: Oxford.

Lewis, D. K. (1986), *On the Plurality of Worlds*, Basil Blackwell: Oxford.

Lewis, D. K. (1988), 'What experience teaches', *Proceedings of the Russellian Society* 13: 29–57.

Locke, J. ([1690] 1975), *An Essay Concerning Human Understanding*, ed. P. H. Nidditch, Oxford University Press: Oxford.

Lopes, D. M. (1995), 'Pictorial realism', *The Journal of Aesthetics and Art Criticism* 53: 277–85.

Lopes, D. M. (1996), *Understanding Pictures*, Oxford University Press: Oxford.

Lopes, D. M. (1997), 'Art media and the sense modalities: tactile pictures', *Philosophical Quarterly* 47: 425–40.

Lopes, D. M. (2005), *Sight and Sensibility*, Oxford University Press: Oxford.

Luquet, G.-H. ([1927] 2001), *Children's Drawings*, trans. A. Costall, Free Association Books: London.

Lycan, W. G. (ed.) (1990), *Mind and Cognition*, Basil Blackwell: Oxford.

McDowell, J. (1994), *Mind and World*, Harvard University Press: Cambridge, MA.

McIsaac, H. K. and E. Eich (2002), 'Vantage point in episodic memory', *Psychonomic Bulletin & Review* 9: 146–50.

McLaughlin, B. P. and J. D. Cohen (eds.) (2007), *Contemporary Debates in Philosophy of Mind*, Blackwell: Oxford.

Martin, M. G. F. (1992), 'Perception, concepts, and memory', *Philosophical Review* 101: 745–63.

Martin, M. G. F. (2001), 'Episodic recall as retained acquaintance', in Hoerl and McCormack (2001).

Martin, M. G. F. (2002), 'The transparency of experience', *Mind and Language* 17: 376–425.

Mather, G. (2006), *Foundations of Perception*, Psychology Press: Hove.

Maynard, P. (1997), *The Engine of Visualization: Thinking Through Photography*, Cornell University Press: Ithaca, NY.

Mazard, A., N. Tzourio-Mazoyer, F. Crivello, B. Mazoyer, and E. Mellet (2004), 'A PET meta-analysis of object and spatial mental imagery', in Denis, Mellet, and Kosslyn (2004).

Moran, R. (1994), 'The expression of feeling in imagination', *Philosophical Review* 103: 75–106.

Nanay, B. (ed.) (2010), *Perceiving the World*, Oxford University Press: Oxford.

Nemirow, L. (1990), 'Physicalism and the cognitive role of acquaintance', in Lycan (1990).

Nigro, G. and U. Neisser (1983), 'Point of view in personal memories', *Cognitive Psychology* 15: 467–82.

Noë, A. (2004), *Action in Perception*, MIT Press: Cambridge, MA.

Noordhof, P. (2002), 'Imagining objects and imagining experiences', *Mind and Language*, 17: 426–55.

O'Shaughnessy, B. (2000), *Consciousness and the World*, Clarendon Press: Oxford.

Owens, D. (1996), 'A Lockean theory of memory experience', *Philosophy and Phenomenological Research* 56: 319–32.

Palau i Fabre, J. (1990), *Picasso: Cubism 1907–17*, Ediciones Polígrafa, S.A.: Barcelona.

Panofsky, E. ([1939] 1972), *Studies in Iconology: Humanistic Themes in the Art of the Renaissance* (1st Icon edition), Harper and Row: New York.

Peacocke, C. (1985), 'Imagination, experience, and possibility', in Foster and Robinson (1985).

Peacocke, C. (1987), 'Depiction', *Philosophical Review* 96: 383–410.

Peacocke, C. (1992), *A Study of Concepts*, MIT Press: Cambridge, MA.

Peacocke, C. (2004), *The Realm of Reason*, Oxford University Press: Oxford.

Pendlebury, M. (1986), 'Perceptual representation', *Proceedings of the Aristotelian Society* 87: 91–106.

Perenin, M.-T. and A. Vighetto (1988), 'Optic ataxia: a specific disruption in visuomotor mechanisms', *Brain* 111: 643–74.

Phillips, I. (2010), 'Perceiving temporal properties', *European Journal of Philosophy* 18: 176–202.

Podro, M. (1982), *The Critical Historians of Art*, Yale University Press: New Haven, CT.

Proust, M. ([1920] 1989), *The Guermantes Way*, trans. C. K. Scott Moncrieff and T. Kilmartin, in *Remembrance of Things Past: 2* (Penguin Books reprint), Penguin Books: London.

Pryor, J. (2000), 'The skeptic and the dogmatist', *Noûs* 34: 517–49.

Pylyshyn, Z. W. (1981), 'The imagery debate', in Block (1981).

Pylyshyn, Z. W. (2002a), 'Mental imagery: in search of a theory', *Behavioural and Brain Sciences* 25: 157–37.

Pylyshyn, Z. W. (2002b), 'Is the "imagery debate" over? If so, what was it about?', in Dupoux, Dehane, and Cohen (2002).

Pylyshyn, Z. W. (2006), *Seeing and Visualising* (1st MIT Press paperback edition), MIT Press: Cambridge, MA.

Robinson, J. A. and K. L. Swanson (1993), 'Field and observer modes of remembering', *Memory* 1: 169–84.

Sartwell, C. (1994), 'What pictorial realism is', *British Journal of Aesthetics* 34: 2–12.

Schier, F. (1986), *Deeper into Pictures*, Cambridge University Press: Cambridge.

Searle, J. (1983), *Intentionality: An Essay in the Philosophy of Mind*, Cambridge University Press: Cambridge.

Shepard, R. N. and J. Metzler (1971), 'Mental rotation of three dimensional objects', *Science* 171: 701–3.

Siegel, S. (2006), 'Subject and object in the contents of visual experience', *Philosophical Review* 115: 355–88.

Siegel, S. (2010), 'Do experiences have contents?', in Nanay (2010).

Smith, A. D. (2001), 'Perception and belief', *Philosophy and Phenomenological Research* 62: 283–309.

Surtees, R. S. ([1854] 1981), *Mr. Sponge's Sporting Tour* (R. S. Surtees Society edition), R. S. Surtees Society: Craddock, Devon.

Taylor, C. (1978–9), 'The validity of transcendental arguments', *Proceedings of the Aristotelian Society* 79: 151–65.

Tononi, G. and C. Koch (2008), 'The neural correlates of consciousness: an update', *Annals of the New York Academy of Sciences* 1124: 239–61.

Tootell, R. B. and M. S. Silverman, E. Switkes, and R. L. de Valois (1982), 'Deoxyglucose analysis of retinotopic organization in primate striate cortex', *Science* 218: 902–4.

Travis, C. (2004), 'The silence of the senses', *Mind* 113: 57–94.

Tye, M. (1991), *The Imagery Debate*, MIT Press: Cambridge, MA.

Walden, S. (ed.) (2008), *Photography and Philosophy: Essays on the Pencil of Nature*, Wiley-Blackwell: London.

Walton, K. (1974), 'Are representations symbols?', *The Monist* 58: 236–54; reprinted in Lamarque and Haugom Olsen (2004), to which all page references refer.

Walton, K. L. (1984), 'Transparent pictures: on the nature of photographic realism', *Noûs* 18: 67–82; reprinted in Walton (2008), to which all page references refer.

Walton, K. L. (1990), *Mimesis as Make-Believe*, Harvard University Press: Cambridge, MA.

Walton, K. L. (2008), *Marvelous Images*, Oxford University Press: Oxford.

Willats, J. (1997), *Art and Representation: New Principles in the Analysis of Pictures*, Princeton University Press: Princeton, NJ.

Williams, B. (1973), 'Imagination and the self', in his *Problems of the Self*, Cambridge University Press: Cambridge.

Wollheim, R. (1965), 'On drawing an object', reprinted in Wollheim (1973), to which all page references refer.

Wollheim, R. (1973), *On Art and the Mind*, Allen Lane: London.

Wollheim, R. (1987), *Painting as an Art*, Thames and Hudson: London.

Wollheim, R. (1998), 'On pictorial representation', *The Journal of Aesthetics and Art Criticism* 56: 217–26.

Wollheim, R. (2003), 'In defense of seeing-in', in Hecht, Schwartz, and Atherton (2003).

Yablo, S. (1993), 'Is conceivability a guide to possibility?', *Philosophy and Phenomenological Research* 53: 1–42.

Zatorre, R. J. and A. R. Halpern (2005), 'Mental concerts: musical imagery and auditory cortex', *Neuron* 47: 9–12.

Zeki, S. and A. Bartels (1999), 'Towards a theory of visual consciousness', *Consciousness and Cognition* 8: 225–59.

Zelevansky, L. (ed.) (1992), *Picasso and Braque: A Symposium*, The Museum of Modern Art, New York and Harry N. Abrams: New York.

Index

Abell, C. 132, 136n, 141n, 142, 165n, 167, 174, 176n, 197n
admissibility requirements 81, 82–3, 159n, 179n, 187n
acuity (in vision and visual mental imagery) 104–5, 110, 112, 121–4
Alberti, L. B. 16n, 61, 158n
appearance-contents
  levels of generality 73–7, 162–5, 167–8, 175–6
  and empty perspectives 42–4
  indeterminacies 77–80
  notion introduced 31
  and ways that things stand sensorily from perspectives 40–1, 67
appearances (memorial)
  epistemological standing 199–202
  future-directed counterparts 210
  nature of 199–200, 203–9
appearances (of possibility) 61n, 210n
appearances (sensory)
  and assertion 30
  associated with types of sensations, see appearance-contents
  contents 30, 41–2, 90–3
  crucial to certain distinctively sensory contents 51–2, 56–57, 67
  epistemological standing 200–1
  and expectations of sensory changes 212–14
  and mentality 41–2, 65–6
  perspectivalness 15–16, 60–1
  presentations-as-true 28–30
  veridicality-conditions 31–2
Armstrong, D. M. 1n, 42n
Arnheim, R. 159n
assertion 30, 186–7
ataxia 39–40

Bahn, P. G. 136n
Ball, T. M. 103n
Bantinaki, K. 132n, 141n
Barsalou, L. W. 215n

Bartels, A. 126n
Berkeley, Rt. Rev. G. 24n
Bermúdez, J. L. 90n
Blumson, B. 131n
Bois, Y.-A. 136n
Boynton, G. M. 124n
Braque, G. 136n
Brewer, B. 29n
Broad, C. D. 206, 208n
Budd, M. 15n, 88n, 132, 141, 142n, 152–4, 172
Bunzeck, N. 128n
Burge, T. 30n, 32n, 200–2, 205n

Casati, R. 170n, 172n
Christensen, D. 202n
Clark, A. 40n
Clark, T. J. 80n
Cohen, J. 198n
conceptual content 8–9, 90–3, 187n
  see also language
Conee, E. 48n
Cooke, G. 71–2
cortical magnification 106, 123–4
Cowey, A. 124n
Crane, T. 17n
Crowdey, J. 211
Cubism 80n, 135–7, 145
Cunego, D. 81
Currie, G. 24n, 111n, 194n

Damasio, A. 126n
Debus, D. 204n
demonstratives 35–6, 95
  see also language
Denis, M. 114n
depiction
  analyses of 131–3, 141–2
  notion introduced 131
  relative crudity of concept 137–9
  semantic heterogeneity 133–9
  see also distinctively visual picturing; seeing-in

distinctively sensory contents
  admissibility requirements, *see*
    admissibility requirements
  and complex contents 185–8, 204–5
  gappiness 8, 54–5, 57, 82, 185–7, 204
  as information, *see* information
  indeterminacies 74–80, 162–4,
    183n, 208n
  and language, *see* language,
    and distinctively sensory contents
  mediating between concepts and
    sensory experiences 214–15
  multiperspectival 80–3, 158–60, 187n
  multisensational 80–3, 182–3
  nature of, summarized 3, 58
  perspective-characterizing, nature
    of 56–8
  recognitional capacities 87–90
  sensation-characterizing, nature
    of 53–5
  and showing, *see* showing
  see also distinctively sensory
    representations; subjective
    informativeness; ways for things to
    stand sensorily
distinctively sensory records
  actual and possible counterparts
    204, 210
  causation 191–5
  epistemological aspects 191–2,
    195–203
  past-directed contents 185–8
  quasi-perceptual aspects 191–2, 199
  see also distinctively sensory record★s;
    drawings; photography; sensorily
    preservative causal chains; sensory
    memories
distinctively sensory record★s 188–90,
  192n, 194n, 197n, 205n, 209n
distinctively sensory representations
  ambiguity 181–3
  arguments against the possibility of
    objective 23–6, 41–4, 67–9, 212n
  class of, first introduced 2
  contents, *see* distinctively sensory
    contents
  and linguistic representations, *see*
    language, and distinctively sensory
    contents
  limited to showing sensible items
    16–18, 61

  more or less schematic 72–4, 162–5,
    167–8, 175–6
  nature of their contents,
    summarized 3, 58
  objective 20–2, 64–9
  past-directed, *see* distinctively sensory
    records
  perspectivalness 15–16, 59–61, 68–9
  relative specificity 18–20, 62
  and showing, *see* showing
  source of numerous limitations upon,
    identified 59–64
  subjective 21–2, 23–5, 53–5, 64–9
distinctively sensory showing, *see* showing
  (showing things as standing sensorily
  certain ways)
distinctively visual pictures 140
  see also distinctively visual picturing
distinctively visual picturing
  analyses of, in general 139
  experienced resemblance analyses 151–6
  metaphysically ambitious
    analyses 141–4
  pretence-based analyses 148–51
  recognition-based analyses 144–7
  see also seeing-in
drawings
  epistemological aspects 195–9
Dretske, F. 18n, 19n
Duncan, R. O. 124n
Dürer, A. 158n

Eich, E. 203n
entitlements 200–2
Evans, G. 37–40
experienced resemblance, *see* distinctively
  visual picturing, experienced
  resemblance analyses

Faulkner, P. 202n
Finke, R. A. 102n, 105, 110, 122n
foreshortening (in pictures) 158n
Foster, H. 136n
Frege, G. 49n, 55, 137, 138n
Friedrich, K. D. 177n
Fruchter, A. 78n
Fry, E. F. 17n

Gardner, S. 215n
Giotto 161
Gödel, K. 201

Goodman, N. 76n, 144n
Gregory, D. I. 9n, 59n, 61n, 66n, 68n, 101n, 142n, 210n
Gregory, L. K. 10, 11, 186
Gregory, M. F. 10, 11, 186
Gunther, Y. 90n

Halpern, A. R. 128n
Handy, T. C. 126n
Harman, G. 30n
Haugeland, J. 12n, 131n
Heck Jr., R. G. 18n, 30, 90n, 95n
Hegel, G. W. F. 69n
Hockney, D. 158n
Hopkins, R. 14n, 15n, 18n, 88n, 132, 136n, 141, 142, 152, 153
Hume, D. 214
Husserl, E. 12n, 206, 212–14
Hyman, J. 138n, 144n, 153n, 161n

illusions
    Müller-Lyer 28
    and sensory appearances 28–9
information 11–12, 173–6, 214–16

Kant, I. 215
Karmel, P. 136n
Keefe, R. J. 183n, 186, 189n
Klee, P. 17n
Koch, C. 126n
Koerner, J. L. 177n
Kornblith, H. 202n
Kosslyn, S. M. 99–124
Kraemer, D. J. M. 128n
Krauss, R. 136n
Kripke, S. 6–7
Kulvicki, J. 76n, 131n, 132n, 144n, 167

labelled axes, see perspectives (sensory), labelled axes
language
    aboutness 137–8
    and distinctively sensory contents 1n, 49, 83–7, 89, 93–7, 147
Le Bihan, D. 126n
Leech, J. 210–11
Le Nain, L. 177–83
Lennard, A. 72
Lessing, G. E. 17
Levinson, J. 172n

Lewis, D. K. 3n, 48n, 166n
lifelikeness (of pictures)
    experience of 172–3
    nature of 162–9
    and photography 198n
    some limits, explained 170–1
    trompe l'œil 160, 169–70, 171–2
    and visual information 173–6
Locke, J. 206–7
Lopes, D. M. 76n, 88n, 130, 131n, 133n, 136n, 138n, 145–7, 161n, 165n, 172n, 174n
Luquet, G.-H. 134

Magritte, R. 161
make-believe, see pretence
Marr, D. 134n
Martin, M. G. F. 23, 30n, 67–9, 90n, 91–2, 207–8
Mather, G. 106n
Maynard, P. 196n
Mazard, A. 107n
McDowell, J. 95n, 215
McIsaac, H. K. 203n
memory, see sensory memories
mental rotation experiments 103–4, 109–10, 112–13, 119–20
Meskin, A. 198n, 199n
Metzler, J. 103–4, 120
Michelangelo 81
modal epistemology 210n
    see also appearances (of possibility)
modes of presentation 49–50
    see also subjective informativeness
Moran, R. 24n

Neefs (the elder), P. 158
Neisser, U. 203n
Nemirow, L. 48n
Nigro, G. 203n
Noë, A. 38n, 213
No Lookerless Looks argument
    presented 23–6
    refuted 41–4, 212n
nonconceptual content, see conceptual content
Noordhof, P. 69n

O'Shaughnessy, B. 34n
Owens, D. 207

Palau i Fabre, J. 135n, 136n
Panofsky, E. 132n
Parmigianino 145
Peacocke, C. 15n, 30n, 33, 37n, 39n,
     68n, 88n, 132, 152, 153
Pendlebury, M. 30n
perception (vs. mere sensation)
     and causation 193
     factivity 193
Perenin, M.-T. 40n
perspectivalness, see appearances (sensory),
     perspectivalness; distinctively
     sensory representations,
     perspectivalness; sensory mental
     imagery, perspectivalness explained
perspective (in pictures)
     linear 158
     oblique 158n
perspectives (sensory)
     auditory 33–6
     bundles of contextual features 31–2,
          36–7
     empty 36–40, 42–4, 65–6
     generality of notion 32–3
     occupied 32, 33–6
     occurrence of sensations at 32
     labelled axes 33–6, 37–41
     origins 33–6
     and pictorial contents 159–60
     tactile 43–4
     visual 31–2, 33–6, 37–9
     see also appearance-contents;
          appearances (sensory)
Phillips, I. 34n
photography
     epistemological aspects 195–9, 200–2
Picasso, P. 17, 135–6, 137
pictorialism (about visual mental
     imagery), see sensory mental
     imagery, Kosslyn's pictorialism;
     sensory mental imagery, Pylyshyn's
     non-pictorialism
pictures
     by children 133–5
     distinctively visual 140
     drawings, see drawings
     in fiction 210–11
     lifelike, see lifelikeness (of pictures)
     and multiperspectivality 158–60
     photographs, see photography
     portraits 188–9

portraying visual sensations 177–83
     see also depiction; distinctively visual
          picturing; seeing-in
Podro, M. 69n
portrayal (of sensations) 21–2, 23–5,
     53–5, 64, 67–9, 177–83
     see also distinctively sensory contents,
          sensation-characterising
possible worlds semantics 3n, 5n, 46
pretence, see distinctively visual picturing,
     pretence-based analyses; pictures,
     in fiction
Proust, M. 38n
Pryor, J. 200
Pylyshyn, Z. 99–124

realism (of pictures), see lifelikeness
     (of pictures)
recognition, see distinctively sensory
     contents, recognitional capacities;
     distinctively visual picturing,
     recognition-based analyses; sensory
     memories, related sensory
     phenomena
Reiser, B. J. 103n
Rembrandt 75
resemblance, see distinctively visual
     picturing, experienced resemblance
     analyses
retinotopic visual areas 106
Robinson, J. A. 203n
Rolls, E. T. 124n

Sartwell, C. 160n, 167n
scanning experiments 102–3, 108–9,
     111–12, 118–19, 120
Schier, F. 88n, 145–7, 174, 176n
Searle, J. R. 21n, 42n
seeing-in 151–5
sense (as mode of presentation), see modes
     of presentation
sensorily preservative causal chains 192–5,
     208–9
sensory appearances, see appearances
     (sensory)
sensory memories
     epistemological standing 199–202
     exclusivism 206–7
     external 204–9
     future-directed counterparts 210
     internal 204–9

neurophysiology 126n
observer 203–4, 209
related sensory phenomena 199,
    207–8, 210
role of sensory mental imagery 203–5,
    206n
see also appearances (memorial)
sensory mental imagery
    behavioural evidence 102–5, 114–15,
        118–21
    inner hearings 127–8
    Kosslyn's pictorialism 99–100,
        107–10, 114–15
    neurophysiological evidence 105–7,
        123–4, 124–7
    perspectivalness explained 68–9
    phenomenology 100–2, 116–18
    Pylyshyn's non-pictorialism 99–100,
        110–13, 115–16
    role in sensory memories 203–5, 206n
    see also acuity (in vision and visual
        mental imagery); mental rotation
        experiments; scanning experiments
sensory perspectives, *see* perspectives
    (sensory)
Shepard, R. N. 103–4, 120
showing (scene-showing)
    nature of 51–2
    notion introduced 50–1
    various features of, explained
        59–64, 67–9, 70–90, 117, 127–8
    see also subjective informativeness
showing (showing things as standing
    sensorily certain ways)
    arises from subjectively informative
        modes of presentation 47–50
    different modes 22, 26, 27, 45–6,
        53–8, 64–5
    potentially supports distinctive
        abilities 47–9
    see also subjective informativeness
Siegel, S. 42n, 78n, 213
Silver Studio 162, 165
Smith, A. D. 30n
Sperber, D. 167n
subjective informativeness
    essential to sensory mental
        imagery 115–17, 127–8
    and lifelike pictures 176
    notion introduced 47–50
    and portrayals of sensations 53

and representational media 99, 100,
    124–7, 128, 143–56
Surtees, R. S. 210, 211n
Swanson, K. A. 203n

Taylor, C. 38n
testimony (using pictures) 186–7, 202
theories of content 6–7, 131
    see also information
theories of distinctively sensory
    content 8–13
    see also information
Thompson, W. L. 107n,
    108n, 109n
Tononi, G. 126n
Tootell, R. B. H. 106n
Travis, C. 29n
trompe l'œil, see lifelikeness (of pictures),
    trompe l'œil
Tye, M. 99n, 108n, 109n
types of sensations, *see* ways for things to
    stand sensorily

Verelst, S. (P.) 164–5
veridicality, *see* appearances (sensory),
    veridicality-conditions
Vermeer, J. 161
Victoria and Albert Museum 72n, 75n,
    81n, 83, 158n, 162n, 164n, 178n
Vighetto, A. 40n
visual mental imagery, *see* sensory mental
    imagery

Walton, K. L. 12n, 24n, 130, 132n,
    148–51, 160, 161n, 193–4n, 210
Watteau, J.-A. 83–5, 138,
    183n, 188–90
ways for things to stand sensorily
    familiar and unfamiliar 71–2
    from empty perspectives 25–6, 42–4
    from perspectives 25–6, 40–1, 213–14
    more or less general varieties 72–4
    predicative roles within distinctively
        sensory contents 53–5, 56–7, 58
    sensory appearances associated with,
        see appearance-contents
    those able to feature in distinctively
        sensory contents 50, 94–5
    types of sensations 27, 46, 120, 123
    see also appearance-contents;
        perspectives (sensory)

Willats, J. 134n

Williams, B. 68n

Wilson, D. 167n

Wollheim, R. 21, 76n, 86n, 88n, 132, 151, 154n, 171–2, 177n, 183n

Yablo, S. 30n, 210n

Zapruder, A. 80, 81n

Zatorre, R. J. 128n

Zeki, S. 126n